Contents

Measuring Clinical Outcome in Asthma

A PATIENT-FOCUSED APPROACH

Edited by

Michael G Pearson and Christine E Bucknall

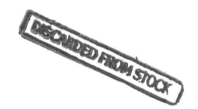

July 1999

Clinical Effectiveness
& Evaluation Unit

ROYAL COLLEGE OF PHYSICIANS

Acknowledgements

The editors acknowledge the contributions of the participants at the meeting upon which the choice of outcome measures described in this document is based, and the staff of the Clinical Effectiveness and Evaluation Unit of the Royal College of Physicians. The costs of the meeting were shared between the RCP Clinical Effectiveness and Evaluation Unit and an educational grant from Glaxo-Wellcome.

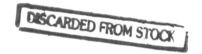
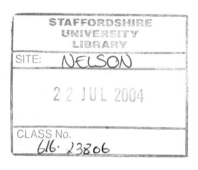
ROYAL COLLEGE OF PHYSICIANS OF LONDON
11 St Andrews Place, London NW1 4LE

Registered Charity No 210508

British Library Cataloguing in Publication Data
A catalogue record for this book is available from the British Library

Copyright © 1999 Royal College of Physicians of London

ISBN 1 86016 097 2

Designed and typeset by the Publications Unit of the Royal College of Physicians

Printed in Great Britain by Sarum Print Limited, Salisbury, Wiltshire

04928501

Foreword

Health professionals are constantly exhorted to prove that the care they provide is effective. This implies the need to measure the outcome of treatment; but measuring outcomes can be quite difficult for chronic medical conditions, like asthma, which vary spontaneously from time to time independent of therapy, and over the years may deteriorate in spite of the very best treatment.

This book describes a process that began with a working party from the Central Health Outcomes Unit (now the National Centre for Health Outcomes Development) which made recommendations for a number of indicators of outcome for asthma. These recommendations formed the basis of a seminar, at which 14 different groups from around the UK came together to pool their experiences using instruments related to patients' experience of asthma. By evaluating the work of the groups, the seminar succeeded in reaching a consensus on three questions to be asked at every asthma consultation to describe the patient's experience. While such a measure of the patient's condition may be less objective than such things as lung function tests, it nevertheless reflects the reality that the patient's description of the effect of their illness is key to evaluating their well-being. Moreover, patients are more likely to listen to their doctor's advice if it is directed towards a goal that they can understand and share.

The British Thoracic Society (BTS), the Royal College of Physicians (RCP) and the National Asthma Campaign in the UK led the way in the development of asthma guidelines that are simple to understand and can be expressed in writing on a single sheet of A4. This simplicity has been highly valued, and goes a long way to explaining the widespread adoption of the guidelines within both primary and secondary care. Similarly, the collaboration on outcome indicators between the RCP Clinical Effectiveness and Evaluation Unit and the BTS is based on the expectation that a simple and straightforward measure of outcome is much more likely to be accepted and used in routine practice.

We are confident that the work described in this book marks a major step towards measuring a clinically important outcome that is relevant to patients. The next step should be to test this measure in clinical practice and investigate how it can be incorporated into NHS information systems. The value of the measurement tool will depend on it becoming part of routinely collected data as part of every consultation, and used to analyse the effectiveness of clinical care.

KGMM ALBERTI
President, Royal College of Physicians

July 1999

Organisations contributing data on patient-focused outcomes

* Authors of papers delivered at the seminar and published in this document

Aintree Chest Centre and Department of Rehabilitation, University of Salford

* Mike Pearson, Director, Clinical Effectiveness and Evaluation Unit,
  Royal College of Physicians of London

Lesley Rimington, Lecturer, Department of Rehabilitation, University of Salford

Blackpool Asthma Care

John F O'Reilly, Consultant Physician, Blackpool Victoria Hospital NHS Trust

Pauline Berry, Nurse, Department of Respiratory Medicine, Blackpool Victoria Hospital NHS Trust

Cornwall Asthma Liaison Nurse Team and Cornwall Asthma Nurse Questionnaire

Ian MacKenzie, Consultant in Public Health Medicine (Primary Care),
Cornwall and Isles of Scilly Health Authority   *Working Group Chair*

Michael Waldron, General Practitioner, Fowey, Cornwall

Department of Public Health Medicine, University of Hull

Jean Peters, School of Health and Related Research, University of Sheffield

Faculty of Human Sciences, University of Plymouth

Michael Hyland, Faculty of Human Sciences, University of Plymouth

Glaxo-Wellcome UK

Rob Pearson, Associate Medical Director, Glaxo-Wellcome UK, Uxbridge, Middlesex

Kathy Cargill, Health Economist, Glaxo-Wellcome UK, Uxbridge, Middlesex

Veronica Prentice, NHS Respiratory Policy Manager, Glaxo-Wellcome UK, Uxbridge, Middlesex

Greenwich Asthma Study

Jonathan Webb, Consultant Physician, Asthma Resource Centre, Greenwich District Hospital, London

Integrated Care: Grampian Asthma Practice Study

J Graham Douglas, Consultant Physician, Aberdeen Royal Infirmary, Scotland   *Working Group Chair*

Liesl Osman, The Chest Clinic, Aberdeen Royal Infirmary, Scotland

Jones Revised Morbidity Index

Kevin Jones, The Medical School, University of Newcastle upon Tyne

National Centre for Health Outcomes Development

* Michael Goldacre, Director, Unit of Health Care Epidemiology, University of Oxford

Alastair Mason, Project Co-ordinator, National Health Outcomes Indicators Project, London

Northampton Asthma Survey

Andrew Jeffrey, Consultant Physician, Northampton General Hospital

Norwich Asthma Control Study

Brian D W Harrison, Consultant Physician (Respiratory Medicine), Norfolk & Norwich Hospital

Yvonne Kelly, Aintree Chest Centre, Fazakerley Hospital, Liverpool

Royal College of Physicians of London

Andrew Georgiou, Research Associate

Salford Asthma Register

Ronan O'Driscoll, Consultant Respiratory Physician, Salford Royal Hospitals NHS Trust, Manchester

Sarah Ansted, Clinical Audit Facilitator, Salford Royal Hospitals NHS Trust, Manchester

Scottish (Tayside) Asthma Management Initiative

Roland Clark, Consultant Chest Physician, Kings Cross Hospital, Dundee, Scotland

Gaylor Hoskins, Tayside Centre for General Practice, Dundee, Scotland

Other contributors to the seminar

* Christine Bucknall, Specialist Registrar, Department of Respiratory Medicine,
Glasgow Royal Infirmary, and Chairman of the Audit Subcommittee of the British Thoracic Society
Standardised Care Committee   *Working Group Chair*

* Duncan Keeley, General Practitioner, Thame, Oxon

Greta Barnes, Director, National Asthma and Respiratory Training Centre, Warwick

J Sandy Bradbrook, Director of AIM 2000, Centre for Health Care Development, Liverpool

Stephen Campbell, Research Associate,
National Primary Care Research and Development Centre, Manchester

H Clague, Consultant Physician, Sunderland Royal Infirmary

Jim Coles, CASPE Research, London

C Kevin Connolly, Consultant Physician, Darlington and Northallerton National Health Service Trusts

Ann Dawson, Consultant Physician, World Health Organisation, c/o DoH, London

Dermot Ryan, Woodbrook Medical Centre, Loughborough

Jonathan Sterne, Senior Lecturer in Medical Statistics,
United Medical and Dental Schools of Guy's and St Thomas's Hospitals, London

Lindsey Taylor, National Asthma Campaign, Providence Place, London

Tim J Williams, Consultant Physician, Kettering General Hospital, Northants

Summary

This publication arises from a project undertaken by the Clinical Effectiveness and Evaluation Unit of the Royal College of Physicians of London leading to an Asthma Outcomes Seminar which investigated the feasibility of reaching a consensus across a national spectrum for a simple patient-focused tool for measuring clinical outcome in chronic persistent asthma. The criteria for the choice of measurement tool were determined from a report by a working group on *Asthma Outcome Indicators* established by the Central Health Outcomes Unit (now the National Centre for Health Outcomes Development) of the Department of Health.

Aims of measurement tools for asthma outcome

The aims of the measurement tool are to:

- reduce or avoid risk of asthma;

- assure return to function after acute asthma attack;

- reduce impact of asthma on general well-being.

Definitions

For an individual asthma patient, the measure is defined by the patient's response to a small set of questions. The indicator is obtained by aggregating results from individuals and expressing them for a given GP, or group of GPs, and divided into age bands for patients.

The project identified 14 different groups from around the country who had worked on the development of instruments that measure patient-focused outcomes for asthma (see page vii). Details about their instruments and data were collected and compared, and all 14 groups participated in a multidisciplinary seminar on Asthma Outcome Indicators held at the Royal College of Physicians on 14 May 1998. This seminar reached complete agreement, after intensive discussion, on the three questions that should be asked routinely at every asthma consultation. The main conclusions from the seminar were:

- Patient-centred outcome measures should be based on genuine symptom outcomes only, excluding any measures of process of care.

- There should be three questions asked at every consultation. These questions should be useful to both clinician and patient and also be a relevant indicator of outcome.

- The three questions, which should cover night-time waking, day-time symptoms and interference with activity, were agreed as:

  In the last week/month

  1. Have you had difficulty sleeping because of your asthma symptoms (including cough)?

  2. Have you had your usual asthma symptoms during the day (cough, wheeze, chest tightness or breathlessness)?

  3. Has your asthma interfered with your usual activities (eg housework, work/school, etc)?

- Each of the above questions should be answerable by a simple *yes/no*, but there could also be supplementary quantitative grades for answers.

This publication includes the presentations to the seminar and reflects the discussions that led to the final consensus. It marks an important step in the development of health outcome indicators for the assessment of levels of morbidity in asthma in both primary and secondary care.

Background and rationale for the choice of outcome indicators

Introduction

Michael G Pearson MB FRCP

Director, Clinical Effectiveness and Evaluation Unit, Royal College of Physicians

In 1993 the Department of Health set up a Clinical Health Outcomes Unit (CHOU — now know as the National Centre for Health Outcomes Development) to look at outcomes in ten medical specialties. I chaired the group on asthma which brought together many different professionals representing different areas of expertise and who were charged with suggesting methods and instruments with which to assess the outcomes of asthma. The findings of the group are expected to be published by the NHS Executive in 1999, along with nine similar reports on other clinical areas.[2]

Asthma was the first topic to be tackled, reflecting the large amount of work already underway in the area including, for example, the development of asthma guidelines by the British Thoracic Society and others, which has in turn spurred on much audit work. This publication follows from the recommendations of the CHOU Working Group on Asthma Outcomes and attempts to pilot, assess and, it is hoped, initiate the use of standardised outcome indicators nationally. The publication is divided into four sections:

1. Discussion of the background to, and rationale for the choice of outcome indicators

2. Papers presented at a seminar on Asthma Outcomes Indicators

3. Summary of the discussion and analysis of the data from the seminar

4. A structured summary of patient-based measurement tools

Background

Recent studies indicate that around 9 million people in the UK have wheezed in the past year and that today over 3 million suffer from asthma.[1] The high prevalence of symptoms has a significant impact on the day-to-day activities of asthma patients and in the past decade there has been a marked increase in the recorded treatment of asthma. The GP consulting rate for asthma increased by 191% between 1983 and 1994/95.[2] The cost to the NHS of asthma, including general practice, hospital inpatient and outpatient care, accident and emergency care and medicines, was estimated at £0.7 billion in 1995/96.[1]

The CHOU Working Group was asked to devise indicators of asthma outcome and, while doing so, to keep in mind the potential uses of outcome information, ie:

▊ Clinical decision-making and audit of clinical work which includes: management of patients; management and audit of health professionals practice and research

▊ Informing decisions about the strategic and operational development of services

▊ Comparison of the organisation for the delivery of service, which could be provider-, purchaser- or population-based

▊ Assessing progress towards standards or targets for health outcomes, agreed locally or nationally, which may be either identified from research literature or set by clinical and managerial decisions

Asthma outcome measurement — summary of points from papers delivered at the seminar

Dr Christine Bucknall's paper, Asthma: the burden of disease, details how asthma is probably the most common disease affecting adults and children in the United Kingdom. There is enormous scope for lessening the burden of asthma through the use of modern inhaled and reasonably safe therapy. It is in this context that patient-based outcome measurements, widely understood and easily collected, can be a valuable guide to applying effective treatment.

Dr Michael Goldacre's presentation, Development of 'ideal indicators' of health outcome: an overview of the Phase III work, described how the outcomes work instigated by the Department of Health advanced proposals about indicators beyond those that are already routinely collected nationally. He described how the impetus for this work was provided by the need to go beyond the traditional use of information about process (eg consultant episodes) and structure (eg number of beds) to consider the *outcomes* of care. As well as asthma, the work covered nine other clinical topic areas: breast cancer, cataract, diabetes mellitus, fractured proximal femur, incontinence, myocardial infarction, normal pregnancy and delivery, stroke, severe mental illness. One of the key aims of the work was to develop indicators that *enhance* measurements and *facilitate* comparison over time and between different places.

In Uses and users of outcome indicators, Dr Bucknall took the discussion a step further by highlighting two perspectives in the field of outcome indicators: the health care professional looking after groups of patients with asthma; and the commissioners of health care who are concerned with the quality of asthma services. Dr Bucknall describes the potential gains from systems of care that promote good practice and enhance systematic assessment of the essential elements of good practice.

Dr Duncan Keeley's presentation, Asthma measurement indices: utility, collectability and applicability to practice, described the enormous potential for outcome measures to achieve real and lasting results. He points out that an outcome measure needs to be *widely used* if it is to improve overall standards of care, and it must serve the perceived needs of both patients and their professional carers. Unless the recommended indicator makes sense to both doctor and patient, it is unlikely to be used.

Health outcome indicators for asthma

When the CHOU Working Group on Asthma Outcome Indicators reviewed the relevant interventions for asthma, it found that there were many different perspectives from which outcomes could be viewed. Moreover, different indicators address different and often discrete parts of the problem. The group therefore devised and adopted a classification using as its model the aims of health care intervention for asthma:

Intention to

- reduce or avoid risk of asthma
- detect asthma early
- reduce or avoid acute attacks

- reduce risk of death

- assure return to function after acute attack

- reduce impact of asthma on general well-being, including the intention to:
  - reduce or avoid complications
  - achieve a target level of lung function
  - improve long-term prognosis

From here the group sought to divide interventions into categories according to whether they were patient-based, clinically based or population-based. For example, a measure of quality of life is likely to be most relevant to the *patient's* perspective, while more immediate *clinical* concerns may focus on measures of pulmonary function. The *population* perspective has a broader view, best addressed by measures able to assess the burden of the disease as a whole. Of course, these perspectives are not necessarily in opposition to each other and are often associated with shared goals. Where possible, the CHOU group sought to develop a set of indicators that would satisfy all three measurement perspectives. The matrix given in Table 1 shows how the 17 different indicators selected by the group relate to these aims and perspectives. The group's report[2] noted that, while some indicators could be implemented immediately, others needed to have further development work carried out on them before implementation could be considered. Of the indicators not ready for immediate implementation, 15A was chosen to be the subject for investigation and development.

Table 1: Matrix to select candidate indicator

Aim of health intervention	Primary measurement perspective		
	Population	Clinical	Patient
▌ Reduce or avoid risk of asthma	1,4		
▌ Detect asthma early		5	
▌ Reduce or avoid acute attacks		2,6,7,8,10,11	15 (A, B & C) 16,17
▌ Reduce risk of death	12,13,14		
▌ Assure return to function after acute attack		3,9,10,11	15 (A, B & C) 16
▌ Reduce impact of asthma on general well-being		2,7,8,10,11	15 (A, B & C) 16,17

Key to indicators

1	Hospital admission rate (PP)	2	Emergency admission rate (PPA)
3	Emergency re-admission rate (PPA)	4	GP consultation rate (PP)
5	GP consultations before diagnosis	6	A&E attendance rate (PPA)
7	BTS Treatment Step profile	8	Incidence of progression to BTS
9	Compliance with BTS guidelines for acute asthma care	10	Current lung function as % of best
11	Loss of best lung function over time	12	Age specific mortality rate
13	Years of life lost	14	Case fatality rate within a defined period
15	Patient assessed impact measures: A. Consultation-based B. Questionnaire-based C. Computer-based	16	Patient satisfaction with asthma care
17	Awareness of asthma management		

(PP) = per general population   (PPA) = per population of people with asthma

Indicator 15A: patient-assessed impact measures

The immediate aim for any doctor is not to improve national statistics but to improve patients' health. Thus, although changes in death rates are of interest, they have relatively little immediate impact on the clinical relationship between patient and doctor. Similarly, most patients are more concerned with whether they feel better, irrespective of the published statistics. Thus, a patient-assessed measure that addresses the aims of reducing or avoiding asthma attacks and reducing impact on general well being is of particular interest. Data are potentially available about symptoms because doctors ask patients questions about their asthma at each clinical contact. However, at present it has not been decided how the data could or should be *collected* and *collated*. This was one of the issues taken up at the seminar. The CHOU Working Group on Asthma Outcome Indicators has specified in its report[2] ways by which these data might be collected including, for example, computerised or routine questionnaires. Each of the different methods has advantages and disadvantages. For example:

■ If information is collected only at a consultation, patients are seen at their worst since many consultations are precipitated by the advent of, or worsening of, asthma symptoms

■ If it is collected from those who attend the surgery or hospital clinic, those who decide not to come constitute 'missing data'

■ If a routine questionnaire is sent out to all asthmatics in a practice, the response rate is likely to be patchy and not representative.

Table 2 provides a more detailed description of indicator 15A.

Basis for planning the seminar on establishing a patient-focused outcome measure

Informal discussions indicated that there were a number of different groups around the UK who had worked on patient-focused outcomes for asthma, and also collected data from a range of routine practice settings and/or through research studies. The questions and structure of the instrument used to assess outcome adopted by the different groups varied considerably. For example, the length of time for which symptoms had been present varied from 1 week to 1 year, and the wording of questions about activity was also quite diverse. The seminar was noteworthy in that it brought together these interested groups from around the country to share their general experiences and explore the possibility of reducing the variation between the different approaches.

Thus, the stated purpose of the seminar was to consider the various outcome measures that had been devised, to compare and contrast them and to see whether it was possible to come up with a degree of *consensus*. The aim was to identify the key information that should be collected by everyone but would also allow those with an individual interest to append other elements to address their particular queries or research need.

Andrew Georgiou from the Clinical Effectiveness and Evaluation Unit of the Royal College of Physicians prepared a digest of the work of the different teams. Section 4 of this publication comprises a more formal version of that digest and includes descriptions of the different indi

Table 2. Indicator 15A

Title

Patient-assessed impact measure: *at consultation*

Intervention aim

Reduce/avoid risk of asthma; assure return to function after acute attack; reduce impact of asthma on general well-being

Characteristics

Specificity: Condition-specific   *Perspective*: Patient

Time frame: Cross-sectional or longitudinal   *Outcome relationship*: Direct

Indicator definition

For an individual asthma patient, the measure is defined by the patient's response to a small set of questions. The following morbidity index revised from Jones *et al* [3] is given as a field-tested example.

Example:
During the past four weeks:

▌ Have you been in a wheezy or asthmatic condition at least once per week?

▌ Have you had time off work or school because of wheeze or asthma?

▌ Have you suffered from attacks of wheezing during the night?

Scoring:
No to all questions = low morbidity; one yes = medium morbidity; more than one yes = high morbidity

The **indicator** would be compiled for a given GP (or group of GPs) and **patient age band** as the response rate mean scores and score profile per practice population of patients with asthma.

Rationale

The questions in this example are sufficiently brief to be used during a consultation as a simple global measure of the patient's assessment of their morbidity. The advantages of the example given are that three of the five areas identified by the working group as particularly relevant for patient assessment are covered (the others are fear as a result of asthma, and impact of asthma on activities beyond school or work). In the example given, the response required is a simple yes or no. There are other examples which prompt the patient for the number of days on which the patient has experienced different symptoms[4] or which refer to a different period, eg a year rather than the last four weeks.

Asthma definition

Asthma as diagnosed by GP (Read code (5 character) H33) and recorded in the patient notes or on an asthma register.

Potential uses

Formal monitoring of these symptoms, with reference to normative data, may be valuable in highlighting the need for alteration in the management of individual cases of asthma, eg appropriateness of medication and organisation of self-care. Aggregated data for this variable could be used for norms, as above; standards for use in local audit (eg within a GP practice); and as a basis for effectiveness comparisons between individual GPs or practices. The validity of such comparisons will be affected by factors including the numbers of cases within the groups being compared, the response rate obtained and the presence of confounding factors.

Potential users

Clinicians, commissioners.

continued

Table 2. continued

Possible confounders

Interpretation of this indicator may be aided if it, and its associated norms, are broken down by British Thoracic Society Treatment Step — acting as a proxy for disease severity. It is also possible that patient assessment of symptoms may vary systematically with age and sex and therefore that consideration should be given to compiling indicators that are age/sex-specific.

Data sources

Self report — verbally. The set of questions would be asked during visits to the surgery and documented in the patient's records. To encourage documentation of this information, these questions could form part of an extended minimum data set for the chronic disease management programme band III.

Data quality

No particular points.

Comments

The focus of the example indicator on the 'last month' represents a sensible compromise between the need for reliability and the limitations of respondents' memories. The indicator could be heavily biased by opportunistic data collection by the GP, ie when the patient presents with what may well be an asthma-related problem. Better data would come from an annual review. As a compromise between these alternatives, data collection could be based around some other regular contact with the surgery, such as the collection of a repeat prescription. As another alternative, stable patients might be targeted for questioning, thus avoiding any patients with a current acute exacerbation of their symptoms. This would, however, entail the reliable identification of stable patients.

cator instruments along with the accompanying data using a review format to describe and assess such factors as their purpose, setting and interpretability.

Each participating team provided a poster display of their experiences and data, and contributed actively to the discussions. There was great enthusiasm and willingness to discuss the generic issues rather than defend individual approaches, and the result was a remarkable and impressive level of agreement.

Reaching a degree of consensus about which data are important to collect is a big step forward and should be of wide interest. We believe this to be the first time that any country has achieved such agreement and that it will have far-reaching implications. For example, computer software houses should be able to incorporate these recommendations into their general practice systems, confident that the most authoritative units in the UK have contributed to and supported the conclusions. If a patient-based outcome indicator can be collected routinely, then the opportunities to use it for improving patient well-being are exciting. With the relevant caveats and cautions about interpretation (described in section 3), the indicator could be aggregated over a practice, a district, or a region, to provide an overall measure of asthma morbidity that would be extremely relevant to an assessment of the health needs of that population.

References

1. Price D, Ryan D. *Asthma: the key facts.* Middlesex: Allen & Hanburys, 1998.

2. National Centre for Health Outcomes Development. *Asthma.* Report of a working group to the Department of Health. London: NCHOD, 1999.

3. Jones KP, Charlton IH, Middleton M, Preece WJ, Hill AP. Targeting asthma care in general practice using a morbidity index. *Br Med J* 1992; **304**: 1353–6.

4. Steen N, Hutchinson A, McColl E *et al.* Development of a symptom-based outcome measure for asthma. *Br Med J* 1994; **309**: 1065–8.

Papers presented at the seminar on asthma outcomes indicators

Asthma: the burden of disease

Christine E Bucknall MD FRCP(Glas) MRCGP

Department of Respiratory Medicine, Glasgow Royal Infirmary; and Chairman, Audit Subcommittee of the Standards of Care Committee, British Thoracic Society

Introduction

Asthma is one of the common chronic medical conditions, with at least 4% of adults and 6% of children having current symptoms.[1] The burden of disease is vast, whether measured in terms of interference with daily life or cost of treatment, both to the patient and to society. Since asthma has also become more common, that burden may also have increased, although more effective treatment and delivery of care are providing a counterbalance.

There are still premature deaths due to asthma, although there is now good evidence of a decline in death rates in the under-65 age group.[1] This is particularly noteworthy in the face of the increasing prevalence of asthma. The recently completed Scottish Confidential Inquiry into Asthma Deaths (SCIAD) suggests that fewer of the deaths that occurred were 'preventable' or, more accurately, associated with adverse management.[2] These observations provide some evidence that the greater recognition of asthma as a chronic condition controllable with long-term medication and the different organisational approach in the UK over the past 10–15 years are beginning to have an impact.

This paper summarises the information on the burden of disease due to asthma in order to set the scene for discussion of patient-based outcome measures, on the premise that knowing the aim or outcome for an individual patient will help to focus attention on the activity needed to achieve it. Health professionals caring for asthma patients have a role in this, but so also do the patients themselves. The evidence from SCIAD is that health professionals have changed practice over the past decade or so.[2] Agreement on significant outcomes will not only provide a further impetus to the process of improving care but also encourage greater patient involvement in the management of their condition.

Number of patients with asthma, and symptom levels

The General Household Survey 1988/89 surveyed a representative sample of households, with all those in the home answering questions (parents answering for those under 16).[1] In the sample of 40,000, 3–4% of adults and 6% of parents responding for children volunteered a diagnosis of asthma in response to the questions 'Do you have a longstanding illness, disability or infirmity?' and, if yes, 'What is the matter with you?' In the under-16 age group asthma was the commonest self-reported illness.

The Health and Lifestyle Survey[3] studied a representative sample of 9,003 adults (aged 18 or over) from households in Great Britain in 1984/85 and 1991/92. There was a marked fall-off in numbers owing to subjects lost to follow-up (including those that had died); only 5,000 were available for the second survey. There was an increase in the self-reporting of asthma, in response to a different style of question from that used in the General Household Survey, with asthma at the top of a list of possible chronic conditions that respondents were asked if they had *ever* had; 9.1% of men and 8.6% of women responded positively in 1991/92. The increase was observed for almost all age groups, taking account of the increase in age of the cohort. Lung function was measured and the decline observed was that expected with age, and there was no increase in the proportion with poor function. However, at the time of the second survey, twice as many respondents were taking bronchodilators or other anti-asthma therapy.

Given that fewer will self-report asthma, compared with the proportion likely to respond positively to a definite question, the percentage of adults with current asthma is likely to be somewhere between 3–4%. For children, the figure is 6% but this may be an underestimate; prevalence surveys of wheeze during the preceding year over the past decade in the UK have consistently found around 12% responding positively.[4]

Many surveys of symptom levels in patients with asthma have been reported, although some of these have described self-selected groups, limiting the wider applicability of their findings. In a community-based survey by Fitzpatrick *et al*[5] which asked about symptoms of sleep disturbance within a larger questionnaire dealing with symptoms of seasonal affective disorder, 6% reported asthma and one-third of these had regular sleep disturbance due to wheeze and also chest tightness on waking in the morning. A similar proportion of parents of children with asthma interviewed in the lifestyle survey reported by Lenney *et al*[4] had waking at night more than once a week during the preceding 12 months. In that survey, carried out by a market research agency specialising in work with children, a representative survey of 773 children with current asthma (and 248 parents of these children) completed questionnaires and interviews. The survey was aimed at children with current symptoms (within the preceding year) *and* a diagnosis of asthma.

Osman *et al*[6] followed patients with asthma attending a hospital clinic who were judged fit for discharge back to their GP. (Chronic severe asthmatics needing continued hospital follow-up were excluded.) Of the control group, 30% reported some restriction of activity, amounting to an average of 7 days per month, in the following year.

The lifestyle survey[4] found that 38% of children interviewed had missed a median 3 days of school owing to asthma in the preceding 3 months, a calculated 10 days per academic year in this group. Hill *et al*[7] recorded 7 days absence per year due to asthma, and Nocon & Booth[8] 6.5 days in the past year. Although some workers have demonstrated a link between consistent absence and poor performance by the end of primary schooling,[9] other studies have found no difference in educational achievement between those with asthma and others.[10,11]

Social and emotional effects

In a qualitative study designed to explore the range of problems associated with having asthma, Nocon & Booth[8] interviewed 18 adults and the parents of 32 children with asthma in Sheffield. They sought to identify a group with current disease, in order to explore the medium- to long-term problems, and used hospital admission a year previously as the means of identifying the study group. Six of the 18 adults had given up work and the others had been off work an average of 22 days in the past year. A total of 36% experienced some restriction of general activities and 43% of school-age children had a degree of difficulty *at most times* with sport or physical activity. The overall social impact correlated with the severity of asthma, categorised by the presence of physical symptoms.

In the above study, 90% of both children and adults felt that asthma had some impact on their emotions: anger, guilt, worry.[8] In another qualitative study, Donnelly *et al* noted that 20% of parents of children with asthma estimated that their child's self-esteem had been diminished because of asthma.[12] A tendency to overprotect children with asthma is reported[4,10] and Donnelly *et al* noted that 52% of parents reported children using asthma to gain attention. In the lifestyle survey,[4] paediatric asthma was noted to have an adverse effect on children's ability to participate in certain sports, play with friends, keep pets and sleep through the night. Just over half (54% of those aged 5–11 and 65% of 12–17 year olds) admitted that they paid less attention than they should at school after a disturbed night. It was reported by 62% of parents that their own social activities were affected by having an asthmatic child, and 70% were constantly aware of their child's asthma.

Asthma may not have only negative effects — some families are brought together by the presence of an asthma sufferer,[8] and in the lifestyle survey[4] two-thirds of parents believed that the presence of an asthmatic child had made other children more kind and understanding. Donnelly *et al* [12] reported that 41% of parents thought their child had become more responsible as a result of having asthma, and 48% thought it made them try harder.

In a National Asthma Campaign (NAC) sponsored poll conducted by Gallup in 1995/96 — in which questionnaires were made available through GPs, pharmacies, supermarkets, national media and via the NAC — 52,000 responses were analysed.[13] More than a quarter of those responding (27%) felt that asthma had a major effect on, or totally controlled, their life; 49% of adults had taken time off work in the preceding year and 71% of children had missed school owing to asthma. The representativeness of this sample must be uncertain but, since two-thirds had seen their GP within the past year compared with data from Morbidity Statistics from General Practice for 1991/92 which suggested that around half of those with asthma consulted with asthma within the year,[14] the data from the NAC poll may be reasonably representative of patients with *current* asthma.

Burden on the community: general practice consultations

The consultation rate for asthma has more than doubled according to data in Morbidity Statistics from General Practice for 1981/82 and 1991/92, with just over 4% of all patients consulting their GP for asthma in 1991/92.[14] The observation that there has been no change in the rate of first episodes of asthma at most ages suggests that increased awareness of the chronic nature of asthma, by both GPs and patients, is responsible for this increase. The weekly returns from general practice to the Royal College of General Practitioners, by which data on a limited range of conditions including asthma are monitored continuously, confirm the upward trend in consultations for asthma, with the incidence of *episodes* of asthma over a 12-week period increasing fivefold from around 10 per 100,000 population in 1976 to 50 per 100,000 in 1994.[1]

Prescriptions

In 1993, asthma prescriptions (an unknown proportion of which will have been prescribed for chronic obstructive pulmonary disease) accounted for 7% of all prescriptions — a net ingredi ent cost of approximately £350 m.[1] The figure for 1995/96 was £511 m.[15] The rate of increase of prescriptions for asthma treatment has been greater than the overall increase, and within the category of asthma drugs there has been a sixfold increase in the number of prescriptions for inhaled corticosteroids. In absolute terms, prescriptions for asthma preparations have increased from around 13 million in 1980 to 33 million in 1993, with about 3 million accounted for by the inclusion of prescriptions from dispensing practices from 1991 onwards.[1]

Hospital admissions

Only a small proportion of adults with asthma are ever admitted to hospital, and the figures relating to hospital admissions are heavily influenced by hospital admissions for children (children under 5 account for a third and those aged 5–14 almost a fifth). Admission rates have risen over the years for the youngest age group, with only a small upward trend for most age groups.[1] Re-admission rates, which account for 10–20% of cases in most series, can be influenced by careful discharge planning and follow-up.[16] In an analysis of direct and indirect costs of asthma from the USA, in which a representative sample of 35,000 subjects reported actual expenditure (the National Medical Expenditure Study[17]), it was observed that 80% of the costs of asthma were incurred by 20% of patients with asthma. Although the actual numbers may be different in the UK, the observation that targeting the care of patients with difficult asthma is likely to have the biggest impact on expenditure, since the cost of hospitalisation is a major influence, is likely to remain valid.

Other costs

Apart from the cost of the drugs used in treatment, an estimate of the cost of other NHS services, except community health costs, for asthma for the year 1989/90 is quoted in a Department of Health overview as a direct cost of £70 m, less than 1% of total costs.[1] This is more likely to be an under- than an over-estimate. Lenney *et al* admit the difficulty of estimating total NHS costs but use data from a number of sources (including consultation costs, prescribed medicines, in- and out-patient care) to estimate the cost of childhood asthma alone at between £78.7 m and £135.5 m (1990).[4]

In 1991/92, well after the introduction of self-certification (which excludes short periods of sickness from the National Insurance scheme, and from official statistics), there were 11 million days of certified incapacity due to asthma. This had risen to 17 million days in 1994/95. Applying the average daily wage for that year of £67,[18] the value for lost productivity is £1,139 m. There has been a disproportionate rise in days lost due to asthma disability, compared with the overall rise in days lost due to incapacity from 1986/87 to 1991/92.[1] Department of Social Security spending on Sickness Benefit due to asthma was £5.5 m and on Invalidity Benefit, payable after 28 weeks absence, was £173.7 m in 1994/95.[19]

Finally, premature deaths due to asthma have a cost, not only in lost productivity but also in human terms. Although death rates are now falling in the UK, and fewer of them are associated with adverse management factors, there is probably still scope for a further reduction in the 1,500 deaths that occur annually in England and Wales.

Conclusion

In summary, asthma is a common chronic disease, probably the most common affecting adults and definitely so for children in the UK. About one-third of these individuals have regular day and night symptoms, and there is a substantial amount of school and other work loss due to asthma. Significant sums of public money are spent on hospital and general practice asthma care, and on benefits claimed because of related incapacity. The information from official statistics is difficult to interpret, although the disproportionate rise in asthma-related incapacity suggests a true increase in asthma disability, rather than employment/ economic effects. Finally, the information from qualitative studies on the emotional impact of asthma, although not all negative, testifies to the wider effects of this common chronic disease. Asthma is largely controllable using modern inhaled and reasonably safe therapy, so there is enormous scope for lessening its burden. The fall in death rates and the lower proportion of deaths involving adverse management factors are the first signs that the changes in asthma care in the UK over the past decade or so are having an impact.

In general management philosophy, the need for setting definite aims and objectives is recognised as an important step towards their achievement. The application of this to asthma management is worthwhile. Agreed patient-based outcome measures that are widely under-stood and easily collectable is the logical next step in applying effective asthma treatment more widely.

References

1. Department of Health. *Asthma: an epidemiological overview.* London: HMSO, 1995.

2. Bucknall CE, Slack R, Godley C *et al.* Scottish Confidential Inquiry into Asthma Deaths 1994–6. *Eur Respir J* 1998; **12**(Suppl 28): 259s–60s.

3. Cox BD, Huppert FA, Whichelow MJ (eds). *The Health and Lifestyle Survey: seven years on.* Aldershot: Dartmouth Publishing Company Ltd, 1993.

4. Lenney W, Wells NEJ, O'Neill BA. The burden of paediatric asthma. *Eur Respir Rev* 1994; **4**: 49–62.

5. Fitzpatrick MF, Martin K, Fossey E *et al.* Snoring, asthma and sleep disturbance in Britain: a community based survey. *Eur Respir J* 1993; **6**: 531–5.

6. Osman LM, Abdalla MI, Beattie JAG *et al* (GRASSIC). Reducing hospital admission through computer supported education for asthma patients. *Br Med J* 1994; **308**: 568–71.

7. Hill R, Williams J, Tattersfield A, Britton J. Change in the use of asthma as a diagnostic label for wheezing illness in schoolchildren. *Br Med J* 1989; **299**: 809.

8. Nocon A, Booth T. The social impact of asthma. *Family Practice* 1991; **8**: 37–41.

9. Douglas JWB, Ross JM. The effects of asthma on primary school performance. *Br J Educ Psychol* 1965; **35**: 28–40.

10. Peckham C, Butler N. A national study of asthma in childhood. *J Epidemiol Community Health* 1978; **32**: 79–85.

11. Martin AJ, Landau LI, Phelan PD. Asthma from childhood at age 21: the patient and his disease. *Br Med J* 1982; **284**: 380–2.

12. Donnelly JE, Donnelly WJ, Thong YH. Parental perceptions and attitudes toward asthma and its treatment: a controlled study. *Soc Sci Med* 1987; **24**: 431–7.

13. Gallup. *The impact of asthma.* Survey results, 1996. London: National Asthma Campaign, 1996.

14. Royal College of General Practitioners, Office of Population Censuses and Surveys and Department of Health. *Morbidity statistics from general practice.* Fourth national study 1991–92. London: HMSO, 1995.

15. Office of Health Economics. *Compendium of health statistics*, 10th edn. London: OHE, 1997.

16. Madge P, McColl J, Paton J. Impact of a nurse-led home management training programme in children admitted to hospital with acute asthma: a randomised controlled trial. *Thorax* 1997; **52**: 223–8.

17. Smith DH, Malone DC, Lawson KA *et al.* A national estimate of the economic costs of asthma. *Am J Respir Crit Care Med* 1997; **156**: 787–93.

18. Office for National Statistics. *New earnings survey: labour market trends.* London: ONS, November 1997.

19. Quoted as personal correspondence, Analytical Services Division, Department of Social Security, Newcastle on Tyne, August 1997 in Price D, Ryan D. *Asthma: the key facts.* Middlesex: Allen & Hanburys, 1998.

Development of 'ideal indicators' of health outcome: overview of the Phase III work

Michael Goldacre BM FSPHM

Director, Unit of Health Care Epidemiology, University of Oxford

This presentation describes how we undertook a project, funded by the Department of Health (DoH), to develop 'ideal indicators' of health outcomes. The DoH had already undertaken work[1,2] to develop health outcome indicators based on routinely available statistical information (notably using mortality data); this represented Phases I and II of the work. Our remit, in Phase III, was to put forward proposals about outcome indicators without constraining our recommendations to data already routinely collected nationally. The background for this was based on the recognition that NHS management makes more use of information about structure (eg availability of beds) and process (eg numbers of finished consultant episodes) than about outcomes. There is also an expectation that the NHS will become increasingly outcome-driven. The 1997 White Paper, *The new NHS*, confirms this.[3] The DoH recognised that outcome indicators are generally not readily available. Where they do exist they have usually been based on data collected routinely for other purposes (eg death certificates). They are therefore *opportunist* rather than *ideal*.

We were asked to undertake work on ten clinical topics; asthma was the first. The other topics, which we have now covered, are stroke, cataract, fractured neck of femur, incontinence, diabetes mellitus, severe mental illness, myocardial infarction, breast cancer, and normal pregnancy and delivery.

The work was undertaken by groups representing a wide variety of perspectives including the views of patients. The different groups included people from clinical practice (nurses and paramedical staff as well as doctors), public health, research, management, and patient groups. The project was led by the Unit of Health Care Epidemiology, University of Oxford, which provided epidemiological input and general co-ordination and used expertise from four support groups:

- The Research Unit (now Clinical Effectiveness and Evaluation Unit) of the Royal College of Physicians for its expertise in setting clinical standards via guidelines and audit

- CASPE Research, London, for its expertise in medical information systems

- The UK Clearing House on Health Outcomes, Nuffield Institute of Health, Leeds University, for its expertise in methods of health outcomes measurement

- The NHS Centre for Reviews and Dissemination, York University, to undertake literature reviews commissioned by the working group

The principles of the health outcomes work were:

- Build on existing work and knowledge

- Establish a structured approach to the development of outcome indicators

▌ Recommend a 'menu' of indicators from which people can choose according to local interests and current concerns

One of the key elements of the work was to emphasise the importance of comparability in indicator measurement in order to:

▌ facilitate comparisons over time and between different places;

▌ facilitate the pooling of data between different departments that want to share data with others;

▌ facilitate the development of 'reference banks' of indicator values that can be used as benchmarks against which to compare information compiled locally.

All these tasks need consistency of concepts, definitions, methods of measurement and methods of comparison.

What do the terms 'health outcomes' and 'indicator' mean?

We defined *health outcomes* as changes (or lack of change when change is expected) in health, health-related status, or risk factors affecting health. A central consideration in this work was that outcomes may be attributable to medical interventions or they may be the result of the natural history of the condition. Considerations of case-mix, bias and confounding are central to the appropriate interpretation of indicator values.

We defined an *indicator* as an aggregated statistical measure, describing a group or whole population, compiled from measures on individuals, that provide insights about the functioning of services. Indicators will not necessarily provide definitive answers on whether services are good, adequate or inadequate but, when well chosen, they should be capable of providing *pointers* as to where further investigation may be worthwhile. We defined *ideal indicators* as what should be known, and realistically could be known, about outcomes relevant to the disease in question.

For each clinical condition, we worked within a model that was developed as an aid to the group to help it identify potential indicators. The model included:

1. an overview of the epidemiology of the disease;

2. the causes and risk factors, the course, and consequences of the condition;

3. relevant interventions.

We considered indicators intended to identify success in:

1. detecting the condition early;

2. reducing the risk of acute attack;

3. assuring return to function after an acute attack;

4. reducing adverse impact on well-being;

5. reducing risk of death.

Under each of these headings we considered possible interventions and indicators of outcome. For each indicator, we devised a structured specification which included the definition of the indicator; the rationale for its use as an outcome indicator; the potential uses and users of the indicator; issues of bias, confounding and interpretation; practical issues of sources of data needed in order to compile the indicator; and other comments and recommendations for further work.

Finally, having worked up the indicator, we specified in the working group report[4] our recommendation for its implementation. We subdivided our recommended indicators into:

- those that in our view should be generally available as a routine;
- those that should be available, where the means to produce them exists locally, or where their production will be possible after expected developments in information technology, or where there is particular local interest in the topic;
- those where, in our view, further work is needed on the technical specification, or the feasibility of data collection, or the usefulness of the indicator before definite recommendations could be made.

For those indicators that we recommended for implementation, we further subdivided our recommendations into those that should be available continuously on a total population basis (eg annual mortality rates for asthma) and those for which periodic availability through sample surveys should be sufficient.

References

1. Department of Health. *Population health outcome indicators for the NHS*. A consultation document. London: DoH, 1993.

2. McColl AJ, Gulliford MC. *Population health outcome indicators for the NHS*. A feasibility study for the Department of Health. London: Faculty of Public Health Medicine of the Royal College of Physicians, 1993.

3. Secretary of State for Health. *The new NHS*. London: Stationery Office, 1997.

4. National Centre for Health Outcomes Development. *Asthma*. Report of a working group to the Department of Health. London: NCHOD, 1999.

Uses and users of outcome indicators

Christine E Bucknall MD FRCP(Glas) MRCGP

Department of Respiratory Medicine, Glasgow Royal Infirmary; and Chairman, Audit Subcommittee of the Standards of Care Committee, British Thoracic Society

This paper outlines the need for outcome indicators, emphasises that outcomes are influenced by many factors, including some over which we have no control, and argues that the various needs of asthma patients, clinicians and commissioners of asthma services can all be accommodated in the interests of good patient care.

In relation to asthma outcome indicators, two different constituencies must be considered — individual patients and groups of individual patients. What is best for the group is not always best for the individual, so there may be some differences in approach, or compromises that are appropriate.

Indicators relevant to the individual

Thinking first of individuals, the aim is to keep them as well as possible on the least possible medication,[1] in order to prevent side-effects. For most patients this should mean the almost complete absence of symptoms and the maintenance of normal lung function, between any exacerbations of asthma that may occur. This requires ways of determining when they are well and when treatment needs to be modified. Increasingly, patients seek this information. The body of evidence for the value of self-management as a tool for keeping patients well more of the time, and at less cost, is growing.[2] Thus, work from Finland has shown a reduction in days of illness, less use of oral corticosteroids, fewer hospital bed days, as well as a cost effectiveness evaluation that indicates how better control can be achieved at a lower cost, both to the patient and to society.[3,4]

Dealing with individual patients involves having one-to-one contact and specifying benchmark indicators of success that are to some extent tailored to the circumstances of the patient. It may be good for one patient to be well enough to dance all night, whereas another may measure success as the ability to go out in the cold morning air to get on with some work. Even this individuality, however, needs to be tempered by the knowledge that most patients with asthma will need to see many different doctors over time. A common goal is therefore more serviceable. This is where the deliberations at the seminar become relevant for the individual patient.

Indicators relevant to groups of patients

Turning now to the needs of groups of patients for outcome indicators, it is useful first to consider the question of who needs to know how groups of patients are progressing. There are two groups here with different perspectives:

- Professionals looking after groups of patients with asthma and running a service in a more or less explicit way

▌ Commissioners of health care, who are likely to be interested in having information on the quality of asthma services

It will be of interest, both to clinicians running a service and to commissioners, to know that patients are 'as well as possible on least medication'. Commissioners are likely also to want comparable data from different units, in order to be able to review the relative effectiveness of different services. However, both clinicians and commissioners share a common interest in good and effective services for asthma patients.

Setting and implementing standards

Effective care for patients with asthma is encapsulated in, rather than dictated by, guidelines. Asthma guidelines have always been based upon available evidence. The evidence base for the UK guidelines has appeared as background papers in *Respiratory Medicine*, both in 1990 at the time of publication of the original guidelines and, more recently, in conjunction with the 1995 position statement.[5–11] The next revision of the guidelines is likely to benefit, at least in part, from formal, up-to-date, systematic reviews. It is now widely recognised that guidelines by themselves do not promote good practice but that their use in a system of care in which systematic review of practice, or audit, is undertaken can improve the quality of care.[12]

Systems of care that remind and prompt clinicians about the key information needed for adequate assessment and thus optimisation of treatment are the keystone of management aimed at keeping patients 'as well as possible on least medication'. It is necessary to combine the merits of having agreed guidelines with the need to remember to use them. Such systems are possible and are in use locally in many places.

There is much to be gained by having widespread agreement about the key information. One possible advantage would be that all GP computer software could be adapted to provide the relevant prompts automatically. Patients would benefit since different doctors and nurses, seen on different occasions, would reinforce similar messages. Clinicians in busy clinical settings would be reminded of the need to do specific things at the right time, and the automation of the data could lead to commissioners having comparable information available to them on the delivery of asthma services.

Examples of applying guidelines in practice

In general practice, Price has shown that systematic assessment of patients, and the greater use of inhaled corticosteroids, was associated with a reduced hospital admission rate, compared with previous experience in the same practice population.[13] Barritt and Staples showed that improvements can be achieved opportunistically, using checklists, booklets and repeated audit.[14] Being systematic about the way in which care is delivered is important: in the work of Connolly *et al* on expressing lung function as a percentage of best function,[15] it was found that the centre in which best function was assessed most rigorously had a higher proportion of its patients within 80% of their best peak expiratory flow (PEF) when stable.

Unfortunately, the evidence for the opposite situation is even more persuasive. Patients who die from asthma have often not been adequately assessed and are often under-treated. They also exhibit personal characteristics, such as greater tendency to poor compliance, which may be less amenable to change. The recently completed Scottish Confidential Inquiry into Asthma Deaths[16] found that patients had fewer adverse management factors, identified by retrospective panel review, than in the 1979 British Thoracic Association study.[17] Nevertheless, at least one such factor existed in 72% of the 95 deaths thought to be attributable to asthma over a three-year period. That study also identifies a decline in the rate of deaths assessed as due to asthma in the 15–64 age group, suggesting that the shift in emphasis to managing asthma as a chronic disease is having an impact.

The delivery of good ambulatory care for patients with asthma is therefore not only intuitively 'a good thing'. Agreed outcome indicators can be used to help ensure that a good standard of care is available for individuals and for groups.

What do outcome indicators tell us?

It is important to remember that the influences of many of the outcome indicators under discussion are not clearly defined and that relatively few of them can be considered as outcomes of health care alone. This is particularly important for commissioners to keep in mind, since clinicians are reminded in everyday practice of the impact of extraneous factors on a patient's possibility of 'a good outcome'.

For hospital asthma management, re-admission rates have now been shown to relate to the quality of preceding hospital care, and can be regarded as a robust outcome indicator.[18]

For ambulatory care, I would argue for the rigorous assessment of best function and expression of stable lung function as a percentage of the patient's best[15] as the prime outcome indicator, or benchmark, both for the individual and for groups of patients. Since this corrects for fixed air-flow obstruction it allows data from groups who may have differing degrees of fixed airflow obstruction to be amalgamated and compared in a meaningful way. It is therefore useful as an outcome indicator for clinicians and commissioners, running and assessing the effectiveness of asthma services, as well as for individual patients.

If most patients (Connolly *et al* propose 80–85% as the target[15]) have stable lung function that is 80% of best, or more, the appropriate secondary target for audit should be the assessment of decline in lung function, over a period of years. This is important since, without knowledge of this, one could not be sure that denominators were not diminishing at an alarming rate without it being recognised. We need more experience before we can define acceptable rates of decline in best function.

If lung function as a percentage of best is less than satisfactory, whether for individuals or groups, further information is needed. This is where some of the other indicators, giving information on current symptoms, use of self-management plans, hospital admission rates and so on, are useful in exploring the reasons for patients being poorly controlled. A staged approach to audit, which ensures that problems can be identified and addressed without the need for continual detailed audit in the face of satisfactory indicators but with mechanisms for investigating unsatisfactory results, can be envisaged.

Everyone can gain from having systems of care in place that promote good practice and reinforce the need for systematic assessment of such practice. Agreement on these essential elements would clarify matters enormously. That was the purpose of the seminar. Patients will have a better understanding of the goals of treatment if professionals agree on these and work towards achieving them in a coherent manner. Clinicians in other specialties gain from systems that remind them of the salient features of good care. Clinicians running asthma services can more easily assess these if there is general agreement on what constitutes effectiveness, and commissioners, spending large sums of scarce resources on the commonest medical condition in the UK, can be more confident when allocating funds.

References

1. British Thoracic Society and others. Guidelines on the management of asthma. *Thorax* 1993; **48**: S1–24.

2. Neville R. Patient education and guided self management plans. *Respir Med* 1996; **90**: 385–6.

3. Lahdensuo A, Haahtela T, Herrala J *et al.* Randomised comparison of guided self management and traditional treatment of asthma over one year. *Br Med J* 1996; **312**: 748–52.

4. Lahdensuo A, Haahtela T, Herrala J *et al.* Randomised comparison of cost effectiveness of guided self management and traditional treatment of asthma in Finland. *Br Med J* 1998; **316**: 1138–9.

5. Barnes PJ. Inhaled glucocorticoids: new developments relevant to the updating of the asthma management guidelines. *Respir Med* 1996; **90**: 379–84.

6. Bosley CM, Corden ZM, Cochrane GM. Psychosocial factors and asthma. *Respir Med* 1996; **90**: 453–7.

7. Bucknall CE. Definitions of severity and outcome measures. *Respir Med* 1996; **90**: 447–52.

8. Clough JB. Recommendations for peak flow monitoring in children. *Respir Med* 1996; *90*: 459–61.

9. Durham ST. Allergen avoidance measures. *Respir Med* 1996; **90**: 441–5.

10. Holgate ST. Inhaled sodium cromoglycate. *Respir Med* 1996; **90**: 387–90.

11. Holgate ST. The efficacy and therapeutic position of nedocromil sodium. *Respir Med* 1996; **90**: 391–4.

12. Grimshaw JM, Russell IT. Achieving health gain through clinical guidelines. II: Ensuring guidelines change medical practice. *Qual Health Care* 1994; **3**: 45–52.

13. Price DB. Patterns of prescribing of inhaled steroids over a seven year period in a general practice and its implications. *Thorax* 1995; **50**: 443P.

14. Barritt PW, Staples EB. Measuring success in asthma care : a repeat audit. *Br J Gen Pract* 1991; **41**: 232–6.

15. Connolly CK, Prescott RJ, Alcock SM, Gatnash AA. Actual over best function as an outcome measure in asthma. *Respir Med* 1994; **88**: 453–9.

16. Bucknall CE, Slack R, Godley C *et al.* Scottish Confidential Inquiry into Asthma Deaths 1994–6. *Eur Respir J* 1998; **12**(Suppl 28): 259s–60s.

17. British Thoracic Association. Death from asthma in two regions of England. *Br Med J* 1982; **285**: 1251–5.

18. Slack R, Bucknall CE. Readmission rates are associated with differences in the process of care in acute asthma. *Qual Health Care* 1997; **6**: 194–8.

Asthma measurement indices:
utility, collectability and applicability to practice

Duncan Keeley MB MRCP DRCOG MRCGP DCH

General Practitioner, Thame, Oxon

This contribution aims to speak for the average general practitioner who is not especially interested in asthma and wishes it would all go away. Whatever is done has to be meaningful for such GPs, as well as for the enthusiasts. This paper relates to the candidate indicator for patient-assessed impact measure at consultation, and begins with an afterthought which comes from the closing lines of a recent article about asthma outcomes analysis:[1]

> *Future work in outcomes should include educating physicians and implementing collection of outcomes data in their everyday practice and the development of easy to use methods of outcomes data collection in the busy office setting ... After all, the ultimate goal of outcomes research is to improve the care of the patient with asthma.*

This is the direction in which we need to go. Whatever else we do and whatever other sophisticated research is undertaken, we need to carry out work on outcomes. Some people at the seminar have been doing it, so we have a basis to work on.

Utility for whom?

Instruments for the compilation of indicators are devised primarily for two groups (see Table 1).

Table 1. The two groups for whom instruments are devised

Group A	▌ Patients
	▌ Nurses/doctors as individual patient carers
Group B	▌ Clinical and health services researchers
	▌ Organised providers of care in hospital and general practice
	▌ Purchasers: health authorities, primary care groups
	▌ Insurance companies
	▌ Managed care organisations
	▌ Pharmaceutical companies
	▌ Government

Group A have to collect the outcomes information
Group B are the main drivers of the outcomes measurement industry
Group A sometimes suspect the motives of Group B

Those in group B are the main drivers of the outcomes measurement industry, but they are not the people who have to collect the data, which is why they may be distrusted by the others and seem to be making their lives difficult with even more work. Suspicions that people have about control and about financial issues and other matters must be taken into account.

I have three short propositions about outcome measures in asthma:

- Asthma outcomes researchers are more interested in asthma than the average health care professional.

- An outcome measure needs to be widely used if it is to improve overall standards of care.

- No outcome measure that fails to serve the immediately perceived needs of patients and their professional carers will be widely used.

As an ideal objective, the business of collecting the indicator must be clear to every doctor and every patient, each time they meet.

What are the needs of patients and professionals?

Table 2. A summary of patient and professional needs

- Both patients and their carers want the asthma to get better.
- Many patients and carers want consultations to be over with quickly.
- 'Fuss minimisation' in health care is a major perceived need of many patients with asthma.
- If asked non-specific questions, patients deny or minimise symptoms so as to avoid being given steroids, and education.

It is self-evident that both patients and their carers want the asthma to get better. Similarly, many patients and carers, as well as doctors, want consultations to be over with quickly. The minimisation of medical care is a major perceived need of many patients with asthma but, if patients are asked non-specific questions such as 'How's your asthma?', they will deny or minimise symptoms because they want to avoid being given steroids, and education, which is what they will get when they tell us, so there may be a disparity between the doctor's perception of an asthma patient and how the patient will respond to a questionnaire such as the asthma audit record cards produced by Allen & Hanburys.

We require a core asthma outcome measure but this is not all we need in looking after a patient with asthma. It is not even what is needed to measure the outcome of asthma treatment, but it *is* a basic nugget of information worth having, to which anything gleaned from a lengthy research questionnaire can be added. What are the attributes of the real nugget — the core asthma outcome measure? It must be *feasible* and *worthwhile* for use in *every* consultation about asthma.

Information captured

The information captured must help to guide individual patient management. It should have a value beyond its worth as an audit tool, because that alone will make people think it is worth collecting. It has to be *short*; three items is the absolute maximum — three bits of information. You must decide who to collect the information from. Other data such as physiological tests can be added as an optional extra. The questions must be based on commonly occurring symptoms which are important to patients, to enable us to find out about hidden or denied symptoms and also because it makes clinical sense to ask about them. By asking patients questions that they perceive to be important to them, it will be found that they do not mind being asked every time they are seen.

There needs to be a sensible standard time-frame for each question. It has to be very simple to put it on a computer, so it must be included in general practice software in a user-friendly manner and formulated in the same way. It also has to be easy to write down because many of us do not bother with computers but prefer a one-line version to use in a Lloyd George record. It has to be interpretable between doctors and nurses, to facilitate sharing of data. It must not involve double entry of information already available from the records in other ways, it must not involve adding up scores because that is too much brain work for a regular activity, and of course it should be reliable, valid and sensitive to change.

Table 3. An example of an abbreviated record.

Record for a reasonably well patient: LM0N LMX0 L3M0D

LM0N = last month no nights disturbed
LMX0 = last month no exercise limitation
L3M0D = no days off in last 3 months

In an example of a shorthand form that might be recorded, the person in the Table 3 illustration has had no symptoms and thus is deemed to be well. All doctors would write this slightly differently, but not very differently, so if there were agreement on something like that there would be the potential for an unprecedented nationwide exercise in routine outcome measurement for an important common illness.

Implementation

Even if no sophisticated analysis is done on the data, the information would still be worth collecting in its own right for use at the simplest level. The information makes sense and is worthwhile even if a practice-level or population-level aggregation of it has not been performed; in many practices I suspect this will not be done easily.

Many data collection methods are possible: at nurse or doctor consultations; through pre-consultation questionnaires; or slipped into repeat prescriptions. The aim is that everywhere patients with asthma are being asked the same three questions, providing doctors and nurses with comparable information.

Standard computer recording is necessary if asthma outcome is to be audited. Incorporation in all GP software packages is necessary to allow standard reporting. So far only remuneration related audit tools have been incorporated as standard into all GP software packages. Maybe what will influence software houses to include something is the possibility that it might be used as part of the general practitioner's remuneration. That is a cynical view, but the immunisation audit and the cervical cytology audit *are* in all the packages. It is not suggested that the chronic disease management regulations should immediately be changed, but GP resentment of data collection requirements would be minimised by decreasing the complexity and maximising the clinical relevance of the data that are requested. Ideally, empirical demonstration of benefit from collecting this information should precede any policy change.

Finally, two problems about aggregation:

1. It is necessary to distinguish between routine and emergency consultations. If the only information is on people having attacks it will look as if everyone is awful. If it is collected only from compliant patients — asthmatics coming to clinics when they are well — it will look as if the data are brilliant. The advantage of asking a question such as 'Yesterday, how many puffs of the blue inhaler did you have?' is that it actually includes something that gives an indication of who is having attacks. The problem is to differentiate between attacks and non-attacks for aggregation.

2. The other big problem is diagnosis and labelling: who has got asthma anyway? What is the denominator? This varies widely between practices. Probably, to aggregate anything meaningful about asthma, the data should be divided between age bands.

Table 4. Attributes of a core asthma outcome measure.

- *Feasible* and *worthwhile* for use in *every* consultation about asthma
- Applicable to people of all ages
- Information captured helps guide individual patient management — not just an audit tool
- Short: three items absolute maximum
- No physiology
- Based on commonly denied symptoms important to patients
- Sensible standard time-frame for each question
- Easy computer recording: user-friendly inclusion in GP software
- Easy paper recording
- No double entry of information already in the records
- No adding up of scores
- Reliable, valid and sensitive to change

Reference

1. Blaiss MS. Outcomes analysis in asthma. *J Am Med Assoc* 1997; **278**: 1874–80.

Health outcome indicators for asthma using patient-assessed impact measures

Andrew Georgiou BA DipLit

Research Associate, Clinical Effectiveness and Evaluation Unit, Royal College of Physicians

The Asthma Outcomes Seminar held in May 1998 at the Royal College of Physicians brought together representatives of teams that have developed instruments for measuring patient-focused asthma outcomes. The occasion offered the opportunity to explore possibilities for reducing the variation between different approaches to data collection and reaching agreement on a single outcome measure for *patient-assessed impact of asthma*. The working group on asthma outcome indicators outlined some of the specifications for such an instrument, stressing that the indicator should be assessed from the patient's perspective. It should also be available to be used either in a cross-sectional time-frame or longitudinally to show improvement or worsening. While the working group provided the example of Kevin Jones' work[1] it also recognised that there were other instruments that had been developed. Some of these instruments are summarised here, highlighting common elements between them as well as the areas of divergence. A more complete review is provided in section 4.

Review format

The template with which each of the instruments was described included:

- *title* of each instrument, listing as reference material background papers, reports etc;

- *purpose* and *setting* of the instrument using the authors' own stated objectives to examine such issues as:
  - who asks the questions (doctor, nurse, postal questionnaire etc);
  - the time-frame (over what period the questions are asked, eg week, month, year);
  - the scoring system (how the answers are valued, measured or scored);

- *interpretation* of the instrument;

- *data and results* from its use in the field or from research studies.

As much as possible this review uses the authors' own descriptions and analysis. It also cites relevant references and reports from where more detailed explanations can be found.

Measurement criteria

The key issues that guided this examination were:

- *Validity*: whether or not the instrument measures what is intended

- *Accuracy and reliability*: inter-rater reliability, repeatability and internal consistency

- *Degree of generalisability*: the ease with which the measure can be used across different conditions, populations and types of investigations

∎ *Applicability and interpretability*: some pragmatic issues, including the administration of the measure, its feasibility, its meaningfulness to the respondent and its ease of completion. The following guidelines have been used:

– The applicability of an outcome measurement assumes a high information value to the practitioner and patient.

– There is not necessarily one single best measure; it may be the case that more than one measure can be used.

– Valid interpretation will also depend on taking into account possible confounding variables such as severity of illness, co-morbidity, case-mix and data quality.

∎ *Responsiveness or sensitivity to change*: the ease with which a measure can be used to detect clinically important change

Similarities in approach

In evaluating the different instruments, a number of identifying *features* and methods of *approach* emerged. Four broad categories of instrument were distinguishable based on either shared characteristics or common background. This is represented by the following table:

A   Jones revised morbidity index

The Short Q Score

Grampian Asthma Practice Study

Faculty of Human Sciences, University of Plymouth

B   Scottish (Tayside) Asthma Management Initiative

Allen & Hanburys Asthma Audit Instrument

Cornwall Asthma Nurse Questionnaire

C   Ambulatory Care Asthma Measure

Northampton Asthma Survey

D   Patient-centred audit tools and registers

Blackpool Asthma Care

Salford Asthma Register

Norwich Asthma Control Study

In group A, the Jones morbidity index is linked to the Hyland (University of Plymouth) work. The work of the Aintree Chest Centre/University of Salford Short Q Score picks up on some of the themes of the Jones work while sharing similarities in approach to the Grampian Asthma Practice Study. The underlying theme behind this grouping remains their simplicity and minimalist approach. They all have the advantage of being pragmatic while seeking to achieve sensitivity to change over time.

The group B family is from the Tayside Asthma Management Initiative which also forms the basis for the Allen & Hanburys work and that of the Cornwall Asthma Task Force. This is a mixed measure containing some direct-impact questions as well as lung function and some process measures. The Tayside stamp is intended to aid the identification of changes of process of care within practices, possibly helping to influence diagnosis and treatment by enhancing co-ordination within the practice.

The symptom-based outcome measure for asthma developed by the Department of Public Health Medicine at Hull is also used by the Northampton Asthma Project (group C). It adopts a *systematic* approach and describes itself as a practical and non-specific measurement tool for audits: patient-centred, multi-domain, and orientated towards outcome and effectiveness.

Group D includes instruments such as Blackpool Asthma Care which provide a patient-centred system for management of asthma patients. As for the Norwich Asthma questionnaire and the Cornwall Asthma Liaison Nurse Team assessment, these are audit tools that review and monitor asthma patient care. The Salford Asthma Register takes this a step forward towards establishing an Information Technology system for the registration, annual review and feedback of data on asthma patients.

This summary of the various instruments highlights an important generic question which is typified best by the different approaches adopted by the Tayside stamp on the one hand and the Jones index on the other. While the Tayside stamp encourages correct process of care with the understanding that improved outcome will follow, the Jones index audits outcome without specifying the processes necessary to achieve the outcome. These variations in approach reflect different aims and approaches to the *dimensions* of health care as described by Avis Donabedian in 1966:[2]

Structure: the availability of suitable buildings, equipment and trained staff

Process: the activities of medical care, eg type of investigation, operation or facilities

Outcome: the change in the patient's current or future health attributable to a medical intervention or other type of antecedent care

These divergences in approach are expressed in the different objectives adopted by the instruments under review.

The Jones index grouping (group A) share a common emphasis on the importance of *simplicity*, as an alternative to *lengthy and time-consuming* questionnaires. They also share Group C's (Ambulatory Care Asthma Measure) stress on the importance of being *practical and condition-specific*.

Alternatively, the Tayside family (group B) and the category of audit tools and registers (group D) emphasise aspects of care that relate to *management and education* of patients (Blackpool Asthma Care) with aims that include *audit facilitation* to help influence patterns of diagnosis and treatment (Tayside Asthma Management Initiative).

While there are differences in approach, it is also important to emphasise the interrelationship between the different dimensions of care. For Hopkins (1990)[3] the process and outcome measures of care are complementary (and not competing) measures of quality. Hence, outcomes are only valid to the extent that they relate to the antecedent process of care, just as measures of the process of care are valid, in so far as they relate to outcome. Generally, outcome measures that are suitable for monitoring health care are required to be simple, straightforward and easily understood, and not too time consuming.[4] But ultimately, in practice it is true to say that the choice of what is measured is dependent on who wants the data, when, and for what reason.[5]

References

1. Jones KP, Charlton IH, Middleton M, Preece WJ, Hill AP. Targeting asthma care in general practice using a morbidity index. *Br Med J* 1992; **304**:1353–6.

2. Donabedian A. Evaluating the quality of medical care. *Millbank Memorial Fund Q* 1966; **44**: Suppl. 166–206

3. Hopkins A. *Measuring the quality of medical care.* London: RCP publications, 1990

4. Hewer RL. Outcome measures in stroke — a British view. *Stroke* Supplement II (1990); **21(9)**: 52.

5. Long A. *Assessing health and social outcomes: Researching the People's Health.* London: Routledge, 1994.

Summary of data and discussion from the seminar on asthma outcome indicators

Discussion points and summary of a seminar on patient focused tools for the clinical measurement of asthma

Prepared by Michael G Pearson MB FRCP

Director, Clinical Effectiveness and Evaluation Unit, Royal College of Physicians

During the seminar a wide range of questions describing patient-based morbidity were discussed. A number of excellent points were made during the day and these are summarised below as a series of questions and discussion. In particular, areas of agreement and disagreement are highlighted as well as issues requiring further investigation/research. The discussion is not referenced partly because many of the references are to the work presented in section 4 of this book, and also because the discussions were more about the general underlying principles than on what has been previously written on this topic.

1. In which clinical context is a patient focused morbidity measure expected to be used?

Age range — There was agreement from the outset that while it was desirable for the proposed outcome indicator to be as relevant to as many asthmatics as possible, it was unrealistic to expect a single outcome indicator to be adequate for both adult and paediatric use. Paediatrics is a whole different area, inviting different measurement criteria, particularly for the under fives. Moreover those present at this seminar were predominantly treating adult patients, and most of the data shown related to adults. So while many of the comments and conclusions may be relevant in paediatrics, the recommendations are intended for those aged 16 and over. It was not considered necessary to consider an upper age limit

Summary note:

The outcome indicator should apply to all patients with asthma aged 16 and over

2. What is a patient-focused morbidity measure?

A patient-focused morbidity measure should not be seen as a substitute to proper diagnosis. This is neither its function nor purpose. Although the questions may also be used by the doctor or nurse when making the diagnosis, the morbidity measure must be clearly seen for what it is — an outcome tool which provides the clinician with information that can indicate the need for more detailed assessment, help target those who should receive extra attention, or in aggregated form, provide information about the overall care in the practice or unit. It is for this reason that the morbidity measure can only be an indicator of outcome rather than a full description of health status.

The key to success of a simple patient-focused morbidity measure will be whether it is perceived as a measure that is *helpful* and that people *want* to collect.

If it is seen as a measure forced upon clinicians through fear of being financially penalised it will not be accepted and generally used. The aim is to establish an outcome measure that is meaningful to clinicians, health service professionals and the patient. The types of uses could be:

▌ to allow practices to distinguish patients requiring extra attention;

▌ to provide comparisons between practices, together with information on prescribing patterns;

▌ to investigate hospital-level care in outpatient clinics.

Summary note:

A patient-focused morbidity measure

is an asthma-specific outcome tool

is not a substitute diagnostic tool

The outcome indicator is to be used only after the diagnosis has been established and should be limited to the most important factors linked to outcome rather than being comprehensive and detailed.

3. Hospital and general practice — Is the patient-focused indicator more relevant to hospital care or general practice?

There was general agreement that whatever indicator was recommended, it needed to be relevant in both primary and secondary care sectors. Although 90% of asthma is managed in primary care, the most difficult and expensive patients attend hospitals as inpatients and outpatients. Ideally, information technology systems should allow data to be shared between hospital and primary care but this may still be some way off in the UK. It is hoped the recommendations of this meeting will prove to be equally useful at all grades of asthma severity.

Summary note:

The indicator should be valid and relevant at all stages of asthma care.

4. What symptoms should the indicator be based upon?

Delegates to the seminar felt it was important that the indicator should be as specific as possible to asthma. This implies that it should be applied only to patients known to have asthma thus establishing an *asthma-specific denominator*. In the early period of use of the measure, where differences relating to diagnostic practice are likely, the denominator may be variable. Increased awareness of, and use of the indicator should in future lead to a greater specificity of diagnosis.

There was much discussion about the appropriateness of including the word 'asthma' in the questions on morbidity. Some participants were concerned that using the word presumes a level of patient knowledge about the full range of symptoms attributable to asthma that may not be justified. Conversely, if the index was to omit the word 'asthma' and phrase a question in the form *'have you had any difficulty sleeping?'*, the answers from patients could become too broad and even include symptoms from many other diseases. Even phrasing a question as *'have you had difficulty sleeping because of a chest problem?'* was felt to be too vague.

Generally, the seminar agreed that the questions should have to specify asthma related problems, understanding that in some cases there is going to be a level of uncertainty and greyness[2]. The actual definition of who has asthma will vary slightly from practice to practice, but because it is an outcome *indicator*, not a precision measurement, it will need to be assessed in conjunction with information on the accuracy of asthma registration. The validity or otherwise of including the word 'asthma' in the questions needs further study.

Summary note:
....

Questions should be as asthma-specific as possible. The indicator is only aimed at one disease and should not attempt to be a generic instrument.

5.   How many questions can an outcome indicator contain?
....

The view expressed by Dr Keeley in his talk, that an indicator must be very simple and straightforward, was echoed many times during the various sessions. A patient morbidity measure has to be something that the GP without a special interest in asthma is going to be willing to use. Much of a GP's work has to be done quickly and thus it must be possible to ask the necessary questions without prolonging the consultation. This implies a simple scoring system that GPs and secondary care doctors can use to obtain an instant snapshot about the individual patient's condition. Ideally it should help indicate whether things are improving, getting worse or remaining stable.

There is an issue of accuracy versus simplicity. A longer questionnaire such as the 72 question St George's Respiratory Questionnaire (SGRQ)[1] has been shown to produce information which has substantial validity as a measure of respiratory health status in a variety of domains. It has been used and proven in many research studies. However, it is not possible to use such a long format in the busy, routine GP surgery. On the other hand, restriction of the instrument to only three questions obviously limits its ability to monitor all aspects of the patient's respiratory health. The instrument becomes less specific and less precise. However, it is possible to ask three questions quickly and to score the answers without prolonging a clinic visit.

If the questions are ones that would or should be asked anyway during a routine consultation, it should be possible to include more questions than if the questions were additional to the routine care of the patient. Some of the presentations in section 4 of this publication refer to comparisons of a three-question score, with various measures of asthma morbidity (symptoms, acute attacks and lung function) and to a four-question (Short Q) score[3] compared to the Juniper Asthma Quality of Life Questionnaire (AQLQ),[4] where there was a strong correlation between the two in 124 patients in four general practices. It is important to recognise however that a correlation between two measures in a group of patients may conceal wide disparities between the two measures in individual subjects — very much the case here since for a given AQLQ score the absolute short Q score may vary by ± 2 points on an 8-point scale.

Nevertheless, the seminar felt that while the number of questions asked (between 3 and 5) was not critical to the success or otherwise of the measure, it is important that the questions are seen to be relevant to the patient's asthma and therefore that the score derived from the questions is reflecting something important about the patient's asthma. In other words, the choice of questions making up the outcome indicator and the context in which they are to be asked is probably more important than the number of questions alone.

Moreover, even if the data collection is to be limited to just three questions, this does not mean the GP has to limit their clinical questioning of the patient. This will continue to be dictated by diagnostic or management need. Similarly, individual practices or hospital units are free to add extra questions as they please to address particular interests or concerns.

The seminar concluded that the final choice of three questions was intuitive as there are no data to show the correct number. The loss of sensitivity and specificity in the individual patient due to restricting the instrument to just three questions is likely to be balanced by the useful comparisons that can be made over time and between different areas using a standard simple instrument. A loss in individual precision is therefore balanced by the gain in overall utility.

Summary note:

It is important that the three core questions comprising the outcome indicator are collected by everybody in a standard and comparable manner. Only then will comparisons between or within practices be possible.

6.   What topics should the questions address?

Five potential topics for questions were apparent from an analysis of the various instruments presented at the meeting (see section 4). These were:

1.   Nocturnal symptoms

2.   Daytime wheeziness

3.   Daytime activities

4.   Use of reliever inhaler

5.   A question about 'bother'

The meeting was unanimous that the first three topics must be included in any score. All the instruments reviewed have questions that fall under these general headings. The use of reliever inhalers has been used in many clinical pharmaceutical trials as a marker of asthma control, the implication being that if a patient needs their reliever inhaler less often, then their asthma is less troublesome. This view was challenged strongly within the meeting. The use of a 'bother' question was also debated but without issue. Each of the five areas is discussed below.

7.   What is the right night time question?

There was complete unanimity that nocturnal wakening because of asthma was a good and reliable marker of poor asthma control. Participants pointed out that although the sleep question appears to be an 'easy' question, it can be misleading for patients who may have a perceived or real difficulty in sleeping, which has nothing to do with asthma. There are also patients who wake for other medical conditions of which prostatism is an obvious example. Thus not only must the clinician be alert to other possible causes of inappropriate answers, but the question to be asked must also be phrased to minimise misunderstandings.

It was noted that the questions asked in the various instruments were all phrased in terms set out by the professions rather than by the patient. If the intention is to ask a patient about sleep disturbance, then it is important to know how patients perceive the question, and whether that perception is different when presented orally or in written form. There is room for some more qualitative research testing patients' interpretations and responses to different questions.

There was considerable discussion about whether to include the word 'asthma' specifically in the question. On one hand it was suggested that if the diagnosis had been made then asthma could be taken as a given, while others argued that the question needed to make it quite explicit that waking from other causes was not part of the enquiry. Without any firm data on this issue, the consensus view was that the question should include the word 'asthma' and, that to be even more specific, the question should make it clear to the patient that cough at night is considered to be an asthma symptom.

Summary note:

The question finally agreed as a result of this discussion was:

In the last week/month 'Have you had difficulty sleeping because of your asthma symptoms (including cough)?'

Further discussion

There was a strong feeling that there should be some degree of quantification of the nocturnal sleep disturbance because many patients may have had one disturbed night which could reasonably be ignored, whereas the physician was really interested in repeated disturbance that would justify a change in therapy.

Quantifying the number of nights in which a patient has woken up at night allows for greater *sensitivity* because it ought to be a measure of *severity*. Moreover it also allows the care of the patient to be audited to check to see if a patient's 'number of nights awoken' has decreased or increased.

8. What about day time symptoms?

There was agreement that it was desirable to ask about the most common and typical asthma symptoms — wheeze, cough and breathlessness. All the various instruments include a day time symptom question in some form.

Summary note:

The seminar agreed there should be a question on day time symptoms in the following form:

In the last week/month 'Have you had your usual asthma symptoms during the day (cough, wheeze, chest tightness or breathlessness)?'

Further discussion

As with the nocturnal question, it was felt necessary to make it quite clear to the patient which asthma symptoms were of concern.

9. Day time activity restriction?

The seminar considered how best to ask a question assessing the impact of asthma on day time activities. Questions asking about how often the patient has taken time off work, are subject to many limitations. First, not all patients have a job or are in full time education. Even those with a job may work for variable periods, so the teacher who is ill during the summer holiday may not record any time off work. Furthermore the concept 'work' can have variable meanings, eg, the effect of asthma on someone whose work involves intensive physical activity is different from someone who works in a less physically strenuous environment.

Various seminar participants emphasised that it was more important to establish whether asthma prevented the patient from doing what they would normally want to do. This is not necessarily measurable in terms of time off work. It was also pointed out that 'days off' is an *exacerbation* question while days bothered is a *control* question — the concepts are different. Days off operationalises better because it is something that people don't want and can understand, ie 'I am too ill to do what I am supposed to be doing – go to work, go to school, do my work'. This is clearly identified with *exacerbation*.

One way of resolving the problem was to phrase the question in terms of activities that the patient would normally do but without specifying that activity in detail. This asks about a change (restriction) in the person's usual activity and in effect allows each individual to act as their own control.

This question makes no assumption as to what a person's normal activity is, but does depend upon what that individual considers to be 'normal' activity. It therefore assesses how much asthma is disturbing the person's lifestyle. Both the housewife, in terms of her ability to get on with her housework irrespective of her asthma, and the office worker who may or may not need to take a day off are included. It also allows the individual patient to control for the type of job that they have. A person who has a sedentary job might continue working but report interference in their overall activity from asthma, whereas the worker in a heavy physical job might have no choice in taking time off; but both would report some restriction of activity.

Summary note:

There should be a question about whether asthma interferes with a patient's lifestyle, in the form:

In the last week/month 'Has your asthma interfered with your usual activities (eg, housework, work/school etc)?'

10. Is beta agonist usage a valid indicator of control?

Although many pharmaceutical studies have used this as an indicator of changing asthma control and one of the instruments (Salford/Aintree Q score) has use of beta agonists as a core question, the seminar was initially very luke-warm about the issue. It was pointed out that the measurement is difficult to perform and its results open to question. For instance, some patients may use their beta agonist very frequently even when their asthma is not bad, either because of habit or anxiety. Second, patients may not remember how often they resorted to beta agonist in the last day or last few days and thus report what they think the doctor 'wants' to hear, and third, effective use is affected by inhaler technique — patients with poor technique will be expected to take more puffs. Lastly, there was a strong feeling that beta agonist use is a surrogate marker and not a primary symptom. It is therefore subject to a lot of 'noise'. The only real support for the concept came from secondary care, since hospital clinicians do not have access to repeat prescription data, which measures the same thing.

Other reasons for rejecting frequency of beta agonist use as an indicator of control were:

▐ Many patients use their bronchodilator on a regular QDS (four times a day) or TDS (three times a day) regime (despite advice in guidelines) and, for such patients, it is difficult to find a phrasing of the question that can distinguish between doses taken for relief of symptoms and doses taken regularly. Moreover, in grouped data there could be enough patients taking their inhalers in this way to obscure any real associations with asthma control. Data (as yet unpublished) were cited from the Salford Hospital study which suggested that there was no association of any other measure of asthma outcome with beta agonist inhaler use when this was assessed by direct question, but there was an association when beta agonist use was measured by recording the number of repeat prescriptions that the patient collected.

- The question becomes invalid when patients are on regular nebulised therapy — which will include many of those with the most severe asthma.

- Since beta agonist prescription data are available on GP computers as a separate but directly collectable measure from the computerised prescription records, it is inappropriate to try and repeat collection of the same data by a separate route. All agreed that repeat prescription data ought to be regularly analysed by GPs and that much useful information could be obtained from such analysis, but this item should be kept separate from the symptom based outcome measure.

Summary note:

Excess beta agonist usage may be important as an indicator of poor asthma control but is better collected from repeat prescription data than by asking the question of patients directly.

11. Should there be a question on 'bother'?

Much of the seminar discussion concentrated on the first questions above and relatively little time was spent on the issue of bother. There are existing studies which attempt to measure such things as the *impact* of asthma on the patient and their *response* to illness. These are totally different domains to those mainly discussed by the seminar, and are worthy of further research and investigation primarily because an important proportion of asthma patients attending hospitals do so out of fear, panic, anxiety and depression, and not just asthma.

The work of Hyland, Cleary and Jones (see section 4) has promoted the concept that a simple bother question incorporates not only the immediate symptoms that a patient experiences but also their ability to cope with those symptoms. Some concern was expressed that a bother question could be confounded by patients who deny symptoms as part of a general denial that they have asthma. However, this could equally well apply to the questions that were retained — a dichotomy that was not clearly resolved. Analysis of the bother question in relation to the Jones morbidity index by Hyland *et al* presented at the seminar, shows that a bother question does produce a different scoring response than the Jones morbidity index. There are patients who are 'high morbidity' on the Jones index who warrant only 'moderate morbidity' on the bother profile suggesting that either the two approaches measure different aspects, or more likely that the threshold of response is different.

The Ambulatory Care Asthma Measure (see section 4) includes a question on 'fear' which also addresses the patient's perception of asthma. These data have so far not been formally analysed and there was concern expressed that those 'poor perceivers' of symptoms who are known to be at greater risk of acute attacks may deny fear. It is not clear if 'fear' is a good or bad indication of control.

Summary note:
....

The meeting did not incorporate a 'bother' question in its final recommendation although the wording of the third question as 'interference' with activity, rather than 'unable to do that activity', implies that the patient is bothered by their asthma.

12. How should the questions be asked to balance simplicity with sensitivity?
....

There was a major issue as to how the three questions should be asked and answered in order to obtain the most useful and reliable answers. The simplest approach is seen in the Jones revised morbidity index which requires a straightforward *yes/no* response and the most complicated in the Ambulatory Care Asthma Measure which requires answers on a five-point scale.

The seminar agreed that the *yes/no* type of response is the one most likely to be used in routine clinical practice. Its very simplicity allows no room for error and adding up the yes answers is easily done without recourse to pen and paper. The data using the Jones revised morbidity index demonstrates that it is an effective tool with which to target patients in general practice who have asthma related problems that are amenable to treatment.[2,6] Such rapid assessment fulfils the requirements of even the busiest practice. Attempts to add more detail would be less likely to achieve consistently reliable results. Jones commented that in an uncontrolled survey in Northumberland, GPs stated that the *yes/no* format was as far as they were prepared to go.

However many participants pointed out that the problem with a simple *yes/no* scoring system is that it lacks *sensitivity*. There are likely to be a range of different responses depending on whether the patient has many or few problems. Experience using the Tayside stamp, with a scoring range for answers of 0 to 3, has shown that it permits treating doctors to recognise a change in an individual, eg, from a score of 3 to 1 for a particular symptom, which under a *yes/no* system could not have been recorded. A graded response to the question on day time activity allows patients to distinguish between having a few minor symptoms and serious difficulty with their asthma — a *yes/no* answer prevents this. Some patients with one minor problem will appear worse due to their tendency to over-report because they are anxious.

In other words, Tayside would argue that their system makes more clinical sense to the people using it, thus enhancing the chance of it being used. The Tayside system has been used in over 3,000 GP practices around Britain, and the Tayside group are not aware of individual GPs finding any difficulty utilising the more complicated scoring system.

Moreover, in secondary care where all patients are likely to have some residual symptoms, a simple *yes/no* answer will set a threshold too low for the tool to be of clinical value — almost all patients will be graded 'high morbidity'. If a three-question tool is ever to be adopted nationally, it has to have utility for, and thus gain support from, both primary and secondary care doctors. A similar problem may apply if the simplest score was applied to the assessment of acute exacerbations — a reason why this indicator is intended for chronic stable asthma care assessment.

Of the various grading systems in use by different units, the four-point score used by Tayside was clearly most favoured and also had the statistical advantage of not having a middle answer, ie it is not prone to a 'middling' tendency as subjects compromise on the central option. However this was not an area discussed in detail and there was insufficient evidence to clearly favour one scoring system over another — an area for further research.

The consensus of the meeting favoured beginning with the simplest form of question and a *yes/no* answer as the basic standard. If such a simple tool could be adopted as a standard measure then much useful progress would have been made. This is because:

- The simpler the tool the greater chance of getting it used in the 'asthma disinterested' parts of the NHS.

- A simple standard does not preclude interested GPs and hospitals from working to the higher standard implied by a graded response system for use within their own practices. They would have necessarily collected and be able to report data for the simpler measure for comparisons with other units.

- Use of a simpler tool as an indicator of outcome, is quite separate from the more detailed questioning which ought to occur as part of every asthma consultation for good asthma management.

- There was no unanimity as to how best to grade the responses except that there should be a similar score system for each of the three questions. The final solution represents a lowest common denominator compromise.

Summary note:

Questions should be asked in order to permit a *yes/no* response about the presence or absence of symptoms. This should form the basic format for all questions. A second level in which those with yes answers are asked a supplementary question about frequency of symptoms requiring a graded answer should be an optional extra.

13. What timescale should be used when asking about symptoms?

Each of the questions should be prefaced with a phrase to the effect of 'In the last week/ month/year' in order to make it quite clear to the patient what time period is to be considered. All were agreed that it would be helpful for the same time period to apply to all three questions to avoid the potential for confusion, but the range of possible time periods ranged from a week to a year.

The problem is to balance the better recollection likely over the previous week against the more representative picture of overall asthma control that can be obtained over a longer period. Asking questions over an annual period is almost certain to run into problems of recall because people will not readily remember time taken off work many months earlier. Conversely, if the time period is made too short, like a day, it may not provide an adequate picture of average severity.

Evaluation trials of the revised Jones Morbidity Index have shown that when the time period for a question was changed from the 'last year' to the 'last four weeks', the levels of statistical association with lung function variables improved. Even the time off work question seemed to have utility over the shorter period. Similarly, a study using the Ambulatory Care Asthma Measure questions over the 'last month' actually correlated very well with all the other health outcome measures looked at. On the other hand the GRASSIC (Grampian) study asked about nights waking per week and days activity per month and days of restricted activity per month, and found that while the nights per week correlated well with many other aspects of asthma control, the same could not be said for the activity question over a longer period (see section 4)

They attributed the worse correlation to people not remembering back accurately for as long as a month. The Salford/Aintree study only used the 'previous week' time period but nevertheless obtained good correlations with the well validated Asthma Quality of Life Questionnaire (see section 4).

One participant of the seminar noted that, given the likelihood of opportunistic data collection, asking about the previous week is much more likely to pick up the effect of any exacerbations, because many consultations will be precipitated by the acute event. On the other hand, if a month were the chosen period, then even in those attending for unscheduled visits precipitated by three or four days of worsening symptoms, the answers ought to reflect the effect of the other 27 days in the month and hence be more representative of background asthma control. This argument holds only if patient recollection is good.

Summary note:
....

It is important to specify the time period that the three questions relate to by prefacing the question with 'in the last week ....' or 'in the last month....' and to use the same time period for all three questions.

The choice of symptoms during the last week or last month needs to be evaluated with further studies.

14. Should the data be collected opportunistically or routinely? — at scheduled or unscheduled visits?

The ideal would be to have the indicator recorded routinely on each asthma patient each year in every practice. However, the workshop recognised that there are many reasons why this ideal is unlikely to be achievable. Some patients may not visit their GP in a given year, some will only be seen when ill, while others will be seen with variable frequency. Defining what comprises a scheduled or unscheduled visit is difficult and might vary according to the mode of organisation in a given practice.

The figures for patients consulting their GP in any one year used to be about 70%. This figure goes up to 90% over five years. The figures have now increased to about 80% in any one year, and 95%+ in the last five years. This would suggest that if information was collected in a consultation-based manner most patients would be included. However, it is clear that not every asthma patient would be included and there are a very small group of patients within the population who are not on any repeat prescriptions, do not consult their GP and do not answer postal questionnaires. A few of these patients may actually be quite ill and ignoring it. But it is likely there will always be a tiny minority who need treatment but who are not directly accessible. It is probably not safe to assume that this group is similar to the attenders. Reference was made to a survey from 1992 which had tried to access a 20% sample of those who had ignored two postal questionnaires and found they had higher morbidity that the main survey cohort.

Summary note:
....

There was a strong view that data should be collected at *each* patient visit to the GP or the practice nurse, whether from scheduled or unscheduled visits. Where possible data from emergency or unscheduled visits should be kept separate from the overall analysis which should attempt to record the underlying background level of asthma control.

15. What is the preferred setting for data collection and who collects the data?

This is linked to the previous question in that the chosen method of collection depends in large measure on whether it is intended to record data at all patient contacts or only at some. There are many issues to be considered relating to data quality and data collectability.

Possible sources of data include GPs, nurses, receptionists (when prescriptions are collected), or pharmacists when patients obtain prescriptions. In addition there is the possibility of postal or even telephone questionnaires.

a **Postal or telephone contacts**

Telephone and postal questionnaires were universally unpopular. Response rates are likely to be variable with no opportunity to control the data quality. Data are therefore likely to be unrepresentative of the true situation and thus not to be taken seriously. Data collected without a face to face interview do not allow the patient to discuss their concerns. The seminar felt strongly that the *human link* in data collection is very important. Postal and telephone methods therefore fail on grounds of collectability, quality and therefore interpretability.

b **Consultation data**

Most of the data presented from previous research studies have been collected through consultation-based questions, either by doctors or nurses. Face to face interviews were strongly favoured as being most likely to obtain reliable data. A computer-based system at a GP practice could be used to prompt the asking of the morbidity measure questions during a consultation. This could also encourage data capture when a patient is visiting a GP for reasons other than their asthma. The practice nurse could also become involved at each patient contact to maximise the number of patients for whom data are available.

Data should be collected at all consultations, but only those for non-acute asthma visits should be entered into the overall analysis. Annual reviews are performed in some practices and should be encouraged but are not comprehensive and should therefore be augmented by data collected during routine visits. The small number of patients receiving asthma therapy who do not attend during a year would have to be contacted in some other way. Although no conclusion was reached on the best way to achieve this, it would clearly be necessary if data are to be comprehensive.

c **Other sources**

Whilst it was recognised that data could be collected by receptionists or by pharmacists at the time prescriptions were collected, there was a feeling that the outcome indicator data really ought to be a responsibility of the medical/nursing team and that patients might feel they were being short-changed if such matters were delegated to receptionists.

There are also problems associated with using pharmacists to collect these data. One of the difficulties is actually retrieving the information from them. There is not, at present, a system for doing this. The other problem is that there is no patient/pharmacist continuity. An asthma patient can visit any number of pharmacies depending on where they are at any one given time. Moreover, some patients pick up their prescriptions at their GP practice, whilst others will have their prescriptions sent to a pharmacist. Finally, it is not always the asthma sufferer who picks up the prescription.

Summary note:

....

The consensus was that the data should be collected every time the patient is seen, but that it should be analysed as an outcome measure for scheduled and not for unscheduled visits. Unscheduled visits imply that the patient is less well controlled. It is worth collecting every time because having the information is useful.

16. The relationship between the primary and secondary care setting?

One of the possibilities for implementing a patient-based morbidity measure suggested during the seminar was an annual review performed by practice nurses but co-ordinated by a hospital-based audit person whose responsibility would be to generate an annual report, after GP validation. Such surveys are certainly possible but would require specific funding, and would not involve primary care using the instrument as part of routine care. There was very limited support for this suggestion from the seminar.

The population of patients in secondary care is very different from that in primary care. Secondary care centres only see 5–10% of asthmatics, although most are at the more severe end of the asthma spectrum. Most of a hospital-based population of asthmatics will have significant symptoms (quite different to that in primary care where many may have no or few symptoms). This may be reflected in the value of measuring symptomatic outcomes. The Beasley and Holgate paper[5] was cited as being able to show a reduction in nocturnal wakenings in a hospital cohort (with data that was normally distributed) but not in primary care (where skewed distributions made interpretation difficult) in response to implementing self management plans. Nevertheless, the seminar was agreed that any instrument had to be useful across the whole spectrum of asthma severity regardless of setting, or it was unlikely to gain acceptance.

It was suggested that it might be better to consider patients by their stage of asthma rather than whether they are being managed in primary or secondary care. The indicator needs to be valid for mild patients and for severe patients regardless of where they are being reviewed. Patients who are symptomatic should have their asthma care reconsidered regardless of where they are in the NHS system.

Doctors treating those with the most severe asthma may well be helped by having the indicator collected using graded answers, to increase the sensitivity of the instrument in assessing change. However, the indicator can still be reported in its most simple *yes/no* format, as well as in a more complex form using graded answers. Secondary care data will be more difficult to compare between centres unless a reliable case severity/casemix variable can be found. However, change over time could be analysed within a centre. Defining the denominator in secondary care will be a challenge.

Summary note:

....

Sharing of data between primary and secondary care is not yet possible on a routine and reliable basis, but the introduction of the promised NHS intranet may make this feasible within a few years. Secondary care patients are likely to need more than questions answered with a simple *yes/no* answer.

17. What is the validity of the proposed measure?

Steen *et al* [7] have published an important paper examining the test/retest validity of their ten question score. The three questions proposed here have substantial overlap with several of their questions. Steen *et al* asked separate questions about cough, wheeze and breathlessness, whereas the proposed question amalgamates the three into a single question under the generic term 'asthma symptoms'. This will need to be tested formally although there are already some data, such as those from the not dissimilar Salford/Aintree Short Q Score (see section 4) to suggest that two week reproducibility is quite good. Unpublished data from the Northampton Asthma Project (see section 4) further suggests that the degree of overlap between the three individual symptom questions in the Steen *et al* format is so great that any one alone might be a reasonably valid surrogate for the others. If confirmed then there should be few problems with a generic asthma question, particularly as it is much closer to the questions that doctors are already asking in real life consultations.

Apart from the consensus achieved, there was a note of caution expressed to the effect that there probably should be some focus group work to ensure that patients do interpret the questions in a consistent manner and that the patient view is similar to that of professionals. Potential problems of translation for those whose first language is not English also need to be formally studied.

Summary note:

The validity and reproducibility of the proposed three question score needs to be formally assessed.

18. How are the data to be used and interpreted?

The definition of the CHOU working group for the patient focused outcome (indicator 15A) was that the indicator would be compiled for a given GP, or group of GPs, and patient age band as the response rate mean scores and score profile per practice population of patients with asthma. This implies that the definition of which patients should be on a GP practice asthma register can be agreed and used uniformly. Most studies suggest that there is a huge difference between practices in their use of asthma registers. This might make it necessary to adopt another less ambiguous definition in the short term — such as patients who are receiving asthma drugs (retrievable from practice computer prescribing) or different levels of asthma treatment.

The value of targeting individual patients who have two or more 'yes' answers has already been described (Jones *et al* [2] and Dickinson *et al* [6]). A further use of the data would be in aggregated form to study variations over time in a single practice or group of practices, or variations between practices or localities. Such comparisons will depend on being able to control for casemix, social class, and deprivation, all of which have been shown to influence the control of asthma. Casemix might be tackled by expressing data separately for patients at different steps of treatment as defined in the guidelines, although this would imply that patients were on the correct treatment step (not always true). It would alert clinicians/managers to potentially incorrect levels of treatment at a practice level.

Aggregated data are less variable than data for individuals but the issue of how data should be aggregated is complex. Adding the answers for the three questions together assumes that the questions are of equal importance. If data are collected using graduated answers on a 0–3 scale there is a further assumption that the points on the scales are equidistant and that the scales for the three variables are equivalent. Such statistical concerns have discouraged the aggregation of data from the Scottish (Tayside) Management Initiative in various publications, but members of the seminar were less inhibited by the statistically purist view and were quite content to aggregate scores for the individual and then to use those scores in overall data for a practice or locality. It is intuitively likely that if the three questions were scored as 0 to 3 and added into a 0 to 9 total, a score of 6 is likely to be associated with worse control than a score of 4. It is possible that this might not be true in all individuals, but in the aggregated data for a practice, reality is likely to be indicated by intuition. This is an area that should be studied further together with the issue of whether gradations should be based on three-, four- or five-point scales of severity.

Many workshop participants expressed the need for caution about using aggregated results at practice level. They felt that these should come with a warning against evaluating the data through simple scores and league tables. They emphasised that there needed to be clarity about the difference between using a patient-based morbidity measure as a tool to look at populations and using it for individuals. There needs to be a very clear statement that looking at these data should also involve looking at the diagnostic criteria of asthma as well as the age and sex breakdown of the practice, deprivation and smoking habits. Recording the BTS treatment step is also an important casemix factor.

As a future perspective, seminar participants heard that if the data were available for practices in a district, then the health authority might use the results to distinguish those practices in the top quartile of morbidity from those in the bottom quartile. These practices might be the ones to be contacted in order to explore the results further. If there was still some residual variation after taking into account all confounding, socio-economic and casemix factors, then we could begin to look into the standard of care provided at practice level. This should not be seen as a policing activity coming from a Health Authority or primary care commissioning group, but rather as a professionally-led exercise in clinical governance. It requires time to *evolve* and be *accepted* by professionals, managers and patients.

At hospital level, most patients will attend for a variable but relatively short period of time while diagnosis is confirmed and then treatment instituted and stabilised. Controlling the data for a changing casemix is therefore essential and it is perhaps doubtful whether useful comparisons can be made because the denominator for a hospital population is indefinite. However, it might be possible to devise systems that would allow before and after scores on outpatients coming through the clinic service, or similar indicators that would provide a guide to the effectiveness or otherwise of the hospital services. More work is needed to assess reliability of a morbidity measure in secondary care assessment.

In all such work it is important to reiterate that the finding that a particular practice or group of practices or hospital unit appear to have worse morbidity data than regional or national averages does not necessarily imply any failure on the part of the clinical team concerned. While there may be a clinical quality failure, apparently poor values might also be due to adverse casemix (confounding by severity) or by an inadequate provision of staff or equipment for the service. A 'poor' result is thus an indicator that further investigation should be undertaken, and not a weapon to castigate health professionals.

Aggregated data may also be useful for comparative assessments of asthma control between practices and localities. Such differences might be the basis for examining populations with 'poor' control to assess both clinical practice and service provision.

Summary note:

How are the data to be used and interpreted?

- ▌ not through simplistic scores of league tables
- ▌ through taking into account age, sex, economic status and casemix
- ▌ must be a professional-led exercise
- ▌ have to be accepted by professionals, managers and patients

SUMMARY POINTS

Agreement was reached on the following three questions:

In the last week/month:

'Have you had difficulty sleeping because of your asthma symptoms (including cough)?'

'Have you had your usual asthma symptoms during the day (cough, wheeze, chest tightness or breathlessness)?'

'Has your asthma interfered with your usual activities (eg, housework, work/school etc)?'

The outcome indicator should apply to all patients with asthma aged 16 and over. It should only be used after diagnosis has been established and limited to the most important factors linked to outcome.

The outcome indicator should be asthma-specific. It should not attempt to be a generic instrument but should be valid and relevant at all stages of asthma.

The three core questions comprising the outcome indicator should be collected in a standard and comparable manner.

The basic format for questions should be a yes/no response about the presence or absence of symptoms. A second level in which those with yes answers are asked a supplementary question about frequency of symptoms requiring a graded answer should be an optional extra.

The choice of symptoms during the last week or last month needs to be evaluated with further studies.

Data should be collected and used as part of the consultation every time the patient is seen, but should be analysed as an outcome measure for scheduled (and not for unscheduled visits).

The data should be used and interpreted:

- ▌ not through simplistic scores or league tables
- ▌ through taking into account age, sex, economic status and casemix
- ▌ must be a professional-led exercise
- ▌ have to be accepted by professionals, managers and patients

References

1. Jones PW. Quality of Life measurement in asthma. *Eur Respir J* 1995; **8**: 885–7

2. Jones KP, Charleton IH, Middleton M, Preece WJ, Hill AP. Targeting asthma care in general practice using a morbidity index. *Br Med J* 1992; **304**: 1353–56

3. Rimington L, Aaronovsky L, Mowatt A, Wharburton E, Ryland I, Pearson MG. Use of a simple patient focused asthma morbidity score. *Eur Respir J* 1997; **10**: 194s

4. Juniper E, Guyatt GH, Epstein RS, Ferrie PJ, Jaeschke R, Hiller TK. Evaluation of impairment of health related quality of life in asthma: development of a questionnaire for use in clinical trials. *Thorax* 1992; **47**: 76–83

5. Beasley R, Cushley M, Holgate ST. A self management plan in the treatment of adult asthma. *Thorax* 1989; **44**: 200–4

6. Dickinson J, Hutton S, Atkin A, Jones K. Reducing asthma morbidity in the community — the effect of a targeted nurse-run asthma clinic in an English general practice. *Respir Med* 1997; **91**:634–40.

7. Steen N, Hutchinson A, McColl E, Eccles MP *et al.* Development of a symptom based outcome measure for asthma. *Br Med J* 1994; **309**: 1065–68

Patient-based measurement tools

1. Jones Revised Morbidity Index (including additional contributions of bother/fright questions)

Papers/reports

1 Jones KP, Bain DJG, Middleton M, Mullee MA. Correlates of asthma morbidity in primary care. *Br Med J* 1992; **304**: 361–4.

2 Jones KP, Charlton IH, Middleton M, Preece WJ, Hill AP. Targeting asthma care in general practice using a morbidity index. *Br Med J* 1992; **304**: 1353–6.

3 Jones K, Cleary R, Hyland M. Predictive value of a simple asthma morbidity index in a general practice population. *Br J Gen Pract* 1999; **49**: 23–6.

4 Dickinson J, Hutton S, Atkin A, Jones K. Reducing asthma morbidity in the community: the effect of a targeted nurse-run asthma clinic in an English general practice. *Respir Med* 1997; **91**: 634–40.

Purpose and setting

The original research (1 above) sought to explore the morbidity of patients diagnosed as asthmatic in general practice; to examine the determinants of this morbidity; and to derive a simple morbidity screening tool for use in primary care. The tool was subsequently used for postal surveillance (2 above) and was then revised (see below) and re-validated (3 above) before being used to show changes following the introduction of pro-active nurse-led asthma care in general practice (4 above). Other research using the index has investigated variations in morbidity patterns between practices (Kevin Jones, personal communication).

Description of original index

Reported morbidity using a calculated index based on three questions:

- Are you in a wheezy or asthmatic condition at least once per week?
- Have you had time off work or school in the past year because of your asthma?
- Do you suffer from attacks of wheezing during the night?

Who asks the questions

The index can be used within a general practice by a GP or by nurses, eg nurse-run asthma clinic. Alternatively, it could be used as part of a postal survey.

Time frame of revised index

In the revised index this has been set as the past 4 weeks.

During *the past 4 weeks*:

- Have you been in a wheezy or asthmatic condition at least once per week?
- Have you had time off work or school because of your asthma?
- Have you suffered from attacks of wheezing during the night?

Scoring system

Scoring:	'No' to all questions	=	low morbidity
	One 'yes'	=	medium morbidity
	Two or three 'yes' answers	=	high morbidity

A possible way to use the index opportunistically in general practice:

LOW morbidity

These patients do not require any further asthma attention for another year.

MEDIUM morbidity

These patients require one dedicated doctor or nurse appointment to assess need for further management.

HIGH morbidity

These patients require full nurse-run clinic assessment and appropriate follow up.

Interpretation

The original and revised indexes appear pragmatically valid in terms of associations with lung function measures (see Tables 1 and 2).

- It is sensitive to change-over time in response to care innovations (see Table 3).

- It seems acceptable as a surveillance tool in general practice.

- It does pick up different spectra of morbidity across samples of practices.

- It may help in the targeting of care to those most in need, provided it is used in conjunction with other measures such as need for hospital admission.

Data collected

Table 1. Lung function variables associated with *original* morbidity index; table first published in 1 above

	Morbidity Index Mean percentage (SD) of predicted values			χ^2	*p*-values
	Low	Medium	High		
FEV$_1$	71.1 (16.4) (n=64)	67.8 (17.7) (n=82)	63.6 (19.7) (n=109)	3.55 * df=2	0.03
Mean peak flow	84.5 (15.6) (n=61)	80.4 (18.8) (n=80)	76.8 (20.3) (n=103)	3.24 * df=2	0.04
Diurnal variation in peak flow	6.9 (5.7) (n=72)	9.7 (7.3) (n=93)	12.4 (8.3) (n=119)	12.62 * df=2	<0.001

* F- ratio (one way analysis of variance)

Table 2. Validity of the *revised* index in terms of lung function; table first published in 3 above

Morbidity index score	n	Mean peak flow as percentage of predicted	Standard deviation
Low	120	91	21
Medium	91	77	21
High	90	63	29

All t-tests performed on these data were significant at $p < 0.001$.

Table 3. Changes in morbidity index, inhaler technique and knowledge scores (n = 173); table from 4 above

Morbidity index score	Initial consultation (number)	6-month review (number)	12-month review (number)
Low	17 (9.8%)	101 (58.4%)	116 (67.1%)
Medium	33 (19.1%)	48 (27.7%)	43 (24.9%)
High	123 (71.1%)	24 (13.9%)	14 (8.1%)

Addendum: Additional contribution of bother/fright questions to the Jones Revised Morbidity Index (work undertaken by Hyland ME, Cleary R, Jones KP)

Papers/reports

1   Jones KP, Bain DJG, Middleton M, Mullee MA. Correlates of asthma morbidity in primary care. *Br Med J* 1992; **304**: 361–4.

2   Jones KP, Charlton IH, Middleton M, Preece WJ, Hill AP. Targeting asthma care in general practice using a morbidity index. *Br Med J* 1992; **304**: 1353–6.

3   Jones K, Cleary R, Hyland M. Predictive value of a simple asthma morbidity index in a general practice population. *Br Med J* 1999; **49**: 23–6.

4   Jones K, Cleary R, Hyland M. Associations between an asthma morbidity index and ideas of fright and bother in a community population. *Respir Med* 1999; **93**: 515–19.

Purpose and setting

There is a need for simple asthma outcome measures for primary care that are valid not only in terms of their relationship with lung function but also in terms of pragmatic psychological constructs. What is the usefulness of adding items on the degree of 'bother' and 'fright' caused by the condition to a previously validated simple asthma morbidity index (Jones revised index)?

Description

As per the Jones revised morbidity index (see above) with the following additions:

▌   During the past 4 weeks, have you felt frightened because of your asthma?

▌   During the past 4 weeks, overall, how much has your asthma bothered you?

Two grading systems were used. One contained three categories: no bother; moderate bother; a lot of bother. The other recorded six categories ranging from no bother to 'makes my life a misery'. For analysis, the six-category version was telescoped into the three categories.

Who asks the questions

This study was carried out through a postal questionnaire survey conducted in one general practice in north-east England.

Time frame

As for the Jones revised morbidity index, ie past 4 weeks

Scoring system

As for the Jones revised morbidity index

Interpretation

Analysis was conducted using simple frequency data with cross-tabulations, correlation coefficients and chi-square values reported as appropriate. Relative risks and confidence intervals were tabled for predictive validity data.

CHAID (CHi-square-Automatic-Interaction-Detection) analysis was conducted to determine whether further segmentation of the morbidity groups, in terms of bother and fright experienced by individuals in the preceding 4 weeks, would identify additional statistically significant associations with adverse events experienced in the preceding 12 months. CHAID is an exploratory decision-tree algorithm that enables the handling of nominal categorical, ordinal categorical and continuous dependent variables. Decision trees are constructed by repeatedly splitting subsets into two or more further subsets, beginning with the entire data set.

The bother question and the Jones index are highly correlated and in many cases provide the same information (see Tables 1–4). However, the bother question as well as the fright question can provide additional predictive information (see Figs 1–3).

Data collected

Responses to the postal questionnaire survey were obtained from 570 individuals; 184 respondents (32%) reported low morbidity, 133 (23%) medium and 253 (44%) high; 29% of respondents had felt frightened by their asthma in the preceding 4 weeks. Both the 'fright' and 'bother' items were significantly associated with the morbidity index.

Table 1. Relative contribution of morbidity index and response to bother question for acute attacks, steroids and more than 4 attacks *(table shows Pearson correlation coefficients, sample size and significance levels)*

	Wheeze at least once per week	Time off work/school	Wheeze during the night	Frightened because of asthma	How much does asthma bother you
Hospitalisation	0.1004 n 761 Sig 0.006	0.1930 n 472 Sig 0.000	0.1728 n 758 Sig 0.000	0.2566 n 748 Sig 0.000	0.2284 n 754 Sig 0.000
Nebulisation	0.1794 n 759 Sig 0.000	0.1585 n 470 Sig 0.000	0.1502 n 756 Sig 0.000	0.2764 n 745 Sig 0.000	0.2563 n 751 Sig 0.000
Steroids	0.2378 n 764 Sig 0.000	0.3059 n 475 Sig 0.000	0.1917 n 760 Sig 0.000	0.3457 n 751 Sig 0.000	0.3788 n 758 Sig 0.000
More than 4 attacks	0.3666 n 756 Sig 0.000	0.2701 n 466 Sig 0.000	0.4057 n 752 Sig 0.000	0.4251 n 743 Sig 0.000	0.4084 n 750 Sig 0.000
Any acute attacks	0.2527 n 752 Sig 0.000	0.2656 n 471 Sig 0.000	0.2260 n 747 Sig 0.000	0.3060 n 738 Sig 0.000	0.3240 n 745 Sig 0.000

Table 2. Acute attacks

	Low morbidity	Medium morbidity	High morbidity
Low bother n/valid responses	8.3% 10/120	10.8% 4/37	20% 5/25
Medium bother n/valid responses	22.5% 10/45	22.6% 19/84	27.9% 41/147
High bother n/valid responses	33% 1/3	40% 4/10	63.2% 43/68

Note: n/valid = number of responses per total number of valid responses, eg 10 low bother answers from 120 valid responses

Table 3 Steroids

	Low morbidity	Medium morbidity	High morbidity
Low bother	12.5%	22.2%	15.4%
n/valid responses	15/119	8/36	4/26
Medium bother	20%	31%	40.9%
n/valid responses	9/45	26/84	61/149
High bother	33%	90%	75%
n/valid responses	1/3	9/10	55/73

Table 4. More than 4 attacks

	Low morbidity	Medium morbidity	High morbidity
Low bother	6.7%	19.4%	34.6%
n/valid responses	8/119	7/36	9/26
Medium bother	22.2%	31.7%	57.4%
n/valid responses	10/45	26/82	85/148
High bother		55.6%	83.6%
n/valid responses		5/9	61/73

Fig 1. Additional contribution of 'Bother' and 'Fright' questions to prediction of patients classified by Jones revised morbidity index: Incidence of any 'acute attacks'

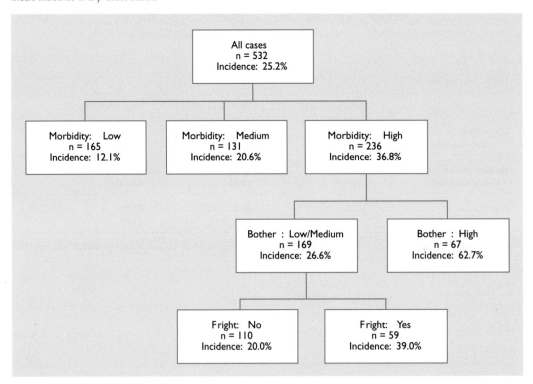

Fig 2. Additional contribution of 'Bother' and 'Fright' questions to prediction of patients classified by Jones revised morbidity index: Incidence of 'more than four attacks'

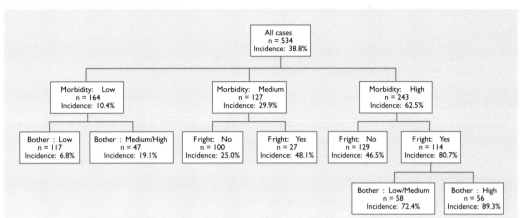

Fig 3. Additional contribution of 'Bother and 'Fright' questions to prediction of patients classified by Jones revised morbidity index: Use of rescue oral steroids

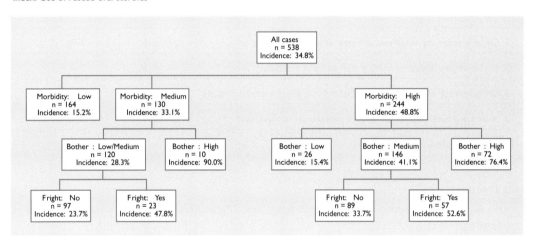

2. Short Q Score

Papers/reports

1   Rimington LD, Aronoffsky A, Mowat A, Warburton E, Ryland I, Pearson MG. Use of a simple patient-focused asthma morbidity score. *Eur Respir J* 1997; **10**: Suppl 25, 194.

Purpose and setting

Effective quality-of-life/symptoms questionnaires (Juniper *et al* 1993, Jones 1992) exist and are validated, but they are too time-consuming and lengthy to include in routine clinical practice.

The Aintree Chest Centre study sought to compare a short (4 questions) score against an established asthma quality-of-life score (AQL) (Juniper). Its aims were to answer the questions:

- How does the Short Q score compare with the AQL score?
- How does our Q score compare with the peak expiratory flow (PEF) score ?
- How does our Q score compare with the level of treatment?

Description

Short Q score

In the past week:	Score	0	1	2
1. On how many days have you wheezed or been breathless?		0–1	2–4	5–7
2. On how many nights have you woken because of asthma?		0–1	2–4	5–7
3. On how many days has asthma prevented you doing normal activities?		0–1	2–4	5–7
4. How many times are you using your reliever inhaler each day?		0–1	2–4	5+

0 = Well controlled   8 = Poor control

Who asks the questions

This study used subjects randomly selected from four GP practices and their asthma registers and included the following:

- Age 16–60 years
- On asthma treatment in past 6 months (repeat prescription for β_2-agonist or inhaled steroid)
- Smoking history <20 pack-years
- No bronchiectasis or previous lung or cardiac disease

The Short Q score is practicable in even the busiest clinic or GP practice. It could be used by any member of a GP practice or hospital clinic, regardless of medical background. The Q score could also be used as part of a telephone or postal survey.

Time frame

The past week

Scoring system

Short Q score

From 0 (well controlled) to 8 (poor control) as described above

Interpretation

■ The Q score correlates well with the established AQLQ (Juniper *et al* 1993) and shows similar relationships to lung function and levels of severity. (See Figs 1–3)

■ The Q score shows sensitivity to changes in asthma status which indicates that it may provide a practical tool with which to estimate asthma morbidity in routine practice.

■ The Q score is short, quick and easy to administer and could be used effectively in a community or hospital based asthma clinic.

■ The Q score has not been tested on a large group of asthma subjects, nor has it been used over a long period of time. Sensitivity to change has not been established.

Data collected

■ Baseline data (age, gender, smoking history, occupation etc)

■ Current medication

■ Spirometry and peak expiratory flow (PEF)

■ Q score

■ Asthma quality-of-life score (Juniper)

■ Hospital anxiety and depression (HAD) scale

Currently 114 patients recruited from four GP practices

Baseline data:

■ Age 42 (±12) years

■ Males 42

■ FEV_1 2.23 (±0.89) litres

■ Predicted FEV_1 3.00 (±0.62) litres

■ PEF 353 (±126) l/min

■ AQLQ symptom score 4.6 (±1.4)

■ Mean total Juniper score 19.03 (±4.9)

■ Mean total Q score 2.74 (±2.41)

■ Mean total HAD anxiety score 8 (±4)

■ Mean total HAD depression score 5 (±4)

■ British Thoracic Society treatment step: 73% steps 1 and 2 (83 patients); 27% steps 3–5

All patients have been followed up over a 2-year period. Data available for publication in 1999. It is hoped that 2-year follow-up data will assess the Q score for reliability and sensitivity over time using comparison with the Juniper AQLQ.

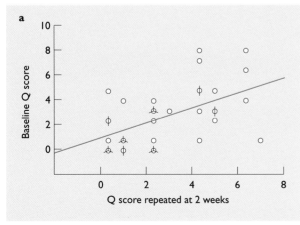

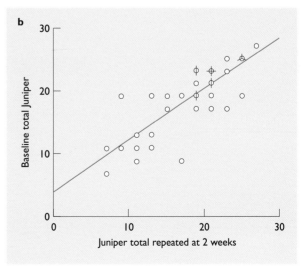

Fig 1. Q score (a) and Juniper (b) show reproducible characteristics.
(a) Rsq = 0.2855; (b) Rsq = 0.6554.

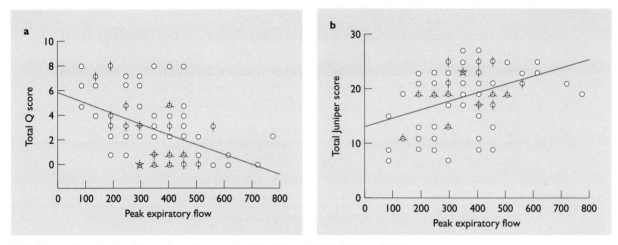

Fig 2. Q score (a) and Juniper (b) correlate with worsening PEF. (a) Rsq = 0.2045; (b) Rsq = 0.1673.

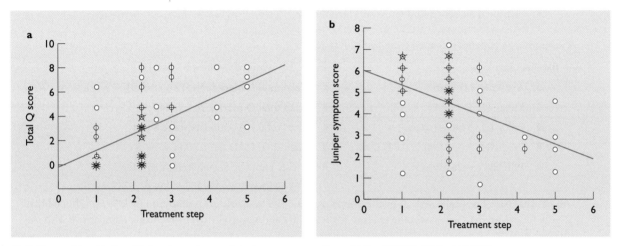

Fig 3: Q score (a) and Juniper (b) show increasing symptoms in more severe asthma. (a) Rsq = 0.2686; (b) Rsq = 0.1817.

3. Cornwall Asthma Liaison Nurse Team

Papers/reports

1   Blackburn LA, Denn DJ, Oliver HF, Vickery PJM, Waldron J. One year's asthma admissions in Cornwall: still deficiencies in basic care. *Thorax*. 1996; **51**: A62.

Purpose and setting

Cornwall's asthma liaison nurses (ALNs) have been in post since April 1995. They are the first community based team of asthma specialist nurses. Each nurse is responsible for all the patients in a specified geographical area. The liaison nurses have developed a form for use when patients are seen during initial consultation and to plan future care. The assessment is intended more as a data collecting method than an outcome tool.

Description

The assessment sheet is made up of sections that deal with:

- Asthma history and medication
- Symptoms past and present
- Assessment including inhaler technique
- Medical management including drug use

Who asks the questions

The ALN's aim is to review all acute admissions at home in the weeks immediately following the hospital stay.

Time frame

Symptoms measured in the past 6 months:

Night/AM	Exercise	Night/AM	Exercise
Never	Rarely	1–2 per week	Hills/stairs
1–2 per month	Running	Daily	Walking on flat

Symptoms that are present now:

- Cough
- Shortness of breath
- Wheeze
- Sputum/vomit

Scoring system

Night/AM		Exercise	
Never	0	Rarely	0
1–2 per month	1	Running	1
1–2 per week	2	Hill/stairs	2
Daily	3	Walking on flat	3

Interpretation

Outcome data reveal that, in a large group of asthmatics sufficiently severe to require hospital admission, there were deficiencies of care in three basic areas:

- Compliance with treatment was unsatisfactory and tended to be worse in smoking households
- Poor inhaler technique is a continuing problem
- Very few patients have any kind of self management plan.

Data collected

In the year April 1995 to March 1996, 521 patients were assessed following admission. This represented 86% of all admissions of Cornish residents with acute asthma.

- 72% had a diagnosis of asthma prior to their admission in the study period
- 42% were less than 5 years of age and 53% were males
- 50% were non-compliant in the use of the prescribed preventer therapy prior to their admission to hospital
- Only 46% of those aged >65 years were non-compliant with prophylaxis compared with 75% of those aged 15–19 years
- 43% of patients had unsatisfactory inhaler technique with their prescribed device
- Only 38% of those aged 15–19 years had poor inhaler technique compared with 60% of those aged >65 years
- Compliance was less good in smoking households
- 94% of patients had no written self-management plan

Assessment

PRE-INTERVENTION — patients assessment

1. Understanding and knowledge of treatment and diagnosis	poor / fair / good
2. Compliance	poor / fair / good
3. Attitude to diagnosis and expectations of treatment	concerns / denial / fear / open / positive

SYMPTOMS (past 6/12)   SYMPTOMS that are present now

NIght / AM		Exercise			Daytime		At night	
					Yes	No	Yes	No
0	Never	0	Rarely	Cough				
1	1–2 per month	1	Running	Shortness of breath				
2	1–2 per week	2	Hill/stairs	Wheeze				
3	Daily	3	Walking on flat	Sputum/vomit				

SCORE   SCORE

LAST ROUTINE ASTHMA REVIEW   EMERGENCY ATTENDANCE(s) THIS EPISODE

(Write in how many times : x)

	Surgery	Asthma clinic	OPD		GP	A&E	In-patient
Never				Never			
<1/ 12				0 – 7.7			
1/12 –3/12				8 – 14/7			
4/12 –6/12				15/7 –1/12			
7/12 –12/12				>1/12 <3/12			
>12/12				COMMENTS			

ACUTE EPISODES IN PAST 6/12 (PRIOR TO THIS ADMISSION)

H = hospital admissions   N = nebulisations   V = visits   S = steroids

The total number of acute attacks is given first and, if wished, the treatment given by the GP can be recorded using H,V,N or S as shown in the notes. For example, if the person with asthma had received 2 visits for acute asthma, a nebulisation at each visit, and on another occasion, when attending the surgery with acute asthma, had received 3 courses of oral steroids, this would be recorded as:

Acute attacks 3
V2 N3 S3

4. Cornwall Asthma Nurse (CAN) Questionnaire

Papers/reports

1   Waldron J, Denn DJ, Oliver HF, Vickery PJM, Waldron MJ, Blackburn LA. *A questionnaire to assess the link between asthma patients' symptoms, their knowledge about management and their feelings about their illness.* Cornwall Healthcare Trust, Asthma Information Centre.

Purpose and setting

The Asthma Liaison Team designed a questionnaire to investigate whether their intervention altered the patients' knowledge, symptoms or feelings about asthma.

Description

The questionnaire covered three key areas:

- The patient's current symptoms
- The patient's knowledge about the appropriate action to take in certain important clinical scenarios
- Patients' feelings about their ability to cope and their level of concern about their asthma

Who asks the questions

The questionnaire (see Table 1) was piloted on 25 patients and then sent to 175 patients seen by the Asthma Liaison Team 2 weeks prior to their first visit, over a 3 month period.

The questionnaire was completed by the patient, or carer in the case of children under 11. For children between 11 and 15 both the carer and the child were asked to complete separate questionnaires. Patients were sent a second questionnaire 3 months later, and a third if they had not responded to the second within a month.

Time Frame

- How often do you suffer from any ASTHMA SYMPTOMS such as coughing, wheeze, breathlessness or chest tightness?
  Every day/ Twice a week or more/ Every couple of weeks/ Once a month; Never

- How often do you WAKE AT NIGHT with any asthma symptoms?
  Every night/ Every other night/ Once a week or more/ Once a month/ Rarely

Scoring system

The patient's current burden, symptoms and their knowledge about important action to take in certain important clinical scenarios is measured by providing tick-box choices.

- Symptom score for night/AM symptoms and exercise:

0	Never	0	Rarely
1	1–2 per month	1	Running
2	1–2 per week	2	Hill/stairs
3	Daily	3	Walking on flat

Inhaler technique: G = good   P = poor
Smoking: Patient   Household
Acute attacks: H = hospital admission   V = visit   N = nebulisation

- Patient feelings about ability to cope were analysed using visual analogue scales, eg

If your asthma was getting worse how would you feel?

0	5	10
not bothered	worried	panicky

Interpretation

The visual analogue scales investigating patient feelings on waking at night, having a bad asthma attack or experiencing worsening asthma symptoms showed highly statistical improvement in all the parameters measured.

Data collected

■ t-tests were carried out on the visual analogue scales that measure patients' feelings of concern on night-time waking, having a bad asthma attack or experiencing worsening asthma symptoms. These tests measured results both before and after intervention. They showed statistically significant improvements after intervention (paired differences 2 tail significance 0.000 to 0.001, 95% CI).

■ However, there was no statistical difference found when looking at the patients' feeling of concern on night waking, or their feelings of concern during worsening asthma episodes. This contrasts with the feelings of the carers who exhibited highly statistically significant improvements in their responses on these parameters.

■ Cornish patients visited by the Asthma Liaison Team are less worried by their asthma symptoms and feel more in control of their disease.

Table 1. The questionnaire includes questions like:

(1)	How often do you suffer from any ASTHMA SYMPTOMS such as coughing, wheeze, breathlessness or chest tightness? *(tick one box only)*	every day twice a week or more every couple of weeks once a month never	❑ ❑ ❑ ❑ ❑
(2)	How often do you WAKE AT NIGHT with asthma symptoms? *(tick one box only)*	every night every other night once a week or more once a month rarely	❑ ❑ ❑ ❑ ❑
(3)	How often do you get asthma symptoms DURING DAILY ACTIVITY such as shopping, home maintenance, playing, housework, sports or child care? *(tick one box only)*	usually often occasionally never	❑ ❑ ❑ ❑
(4)	If you were to WAKE AT NIGHT with symptoms would you IMMEDIATELY .... *(tick any number of boxes)*	do nothing have a drink take your reliever inhaler get some fresh air phone the doctor take your preventer inhaler	❑ ❑ ❑ ❑ ❑ ❑

(5) How would you feel if you were to WAKE AT NIGHT with asthma symptoms?
Mark both lines in the most appropriate place

(a)

0	5	10
not bothered	worried	panicky

(b)

0	5	10
totally in control	able to manage	unable to cope

(6) If you were to have a BAD asthma attack would you: *(tick any number of boxes)*

❑ lie down	❑ take your reliever inhaler	❑ ignore it
❑ sit in a steamy room	❑ seek medical help	❑ keep calm
❑ take your preventer inhaler	❑ do your peak flow	❑ go for a walk

5. Scottish (Tayside) Asthma Management Initiative

Papers/reports

1   Bryce FP, Neville RG, Crombie IK, Clark RA, McKenzie P. Controlled trial of an audit facilitator in diagnosis and treatment of childhood asthma in general practice. *Br Med J* 1995; **310**: 838–42.

2   Duffy R, Neville RG, Hoskins G, Smith B, McCowan C. Who is admitted to hospital with asthma? *Asthma in General Practice* 1997; **5**(1): 5–7. ISSN: 0968-039X.

3   Hoskins G, Neville RG, Smith B, Clark RA. Does participation in distance learning and audit improve the care of patients with acute asthma attacks. *Health Bulletin* 1997; **55**(3): 150–155.

4   Hoskins G, Smith B, Neville RG, Clark RA. The Tayside asthma management initiative. *Health Bulletin* 1998; **56**(2): 586–591.

5   McCowan C, Neville RG, Crombie IK, Clark RA, Warner FC. The facilitator effect: results from a four-year follow-up of children with asthma. *Br J Gen Pract.* 1997; **47**: 156–60.

6   Neville R. Two approaches to effective asthma audit. *Practitioner* 1995; **239**: 203–5.

7   Neville RG, Hoskins G, Smith B, Clark RA. Observations on the structure process and clinical outcomes of asthma care in general practice. *Br J Gen Pract* 1996; **46**: 583–7.

Purpose and setting

A facilitator acts as a catalyst to assist change within practices. This is a method in which practices receive help and advice which affects clinical management of large groups of patients. The use of an audit facilitator can thus have a favourable influence on the pattern of diagnosis and treatment of asthma in general practice.

The Tayside Asthma Assessment Stamp provides an opportunity to ensure that all members of the healthcare team are assessing asthma in a co-ordinated way.

Description

The Clinical Assessment Recording Stamp:

- At-night symptom score (never; 1–2 per month; 1–2 per week; daily)
- On waking symptom score (never; 1–2 per monthly; 1–2 per week; daily)
- Interference of asthma on activity
- PEFR (random measurement on assessment) + % of best
- Compliance (satisfactory; unsatisfactory)
- Inhaler technique (satisfactory; unsatisfactory)
- Days off per month (work; school; leisure)
- Follow-up (number of weeks)
- Reliever medication use in last 24 hours

Who asks the questions

The key to running a successful audit is to involve all practice members from the start in the audit process. An electronic version of the stamp is also available.

The Tayside Asthma Assessment Stamp can act as an aide memoir for important aspects of clinical care. It is quick and easy to use; this is because it is stamp-based and there is no need for extra written materials in case notes. It is also relevant for all patients with chronic asthma. It is quicker to use than conventional note entry during busy clinics. It can be widely used as an assessment tool in primary care. Little teaching is required and it is usable without additional paperwork.

Time frame

At-night symptom score	(daily; weekly; monthly)
On-waking symptom score	(daily; weekly; monthly)

Scoring system

■ At-night symptom score: 0 = never; 1 = 1-2 per month; 2 = 1-2 per week; 3 = daily

■ On-waking symptom score: 0 = never; 1 = 1-2 per month; 2 = 1-2 per week; 3 = daily

■ Exercise or activity: 0 = rarely; 1 = running; 2 = hills/stairs; 3 = walking on flat.

■ Compliance: satisfactory (S); unsatisfactory (U)

■ Inhaler technique: adequate (A); not adequate (N)

Interpretation

The data generated using the stamp can be used to compare individual patient scores from one assessment to the next or to build a picture of the overall quality of asthma care.

■ The scores correlate with a variety of things: night symptom scores correlate with adverse outcome in children; exercise scores with adverse outcome in adults.

■ The scores 0, 1, 2, 3 are nominal, not integral, and thus should not be summated.

Data collected

The Tayside Asthma Assessment Stamp has been used and evaluated as an assessment tool in a variety of national and local studies, eg National Asthma Management Study of 1994–96, Tayside and Fife Asthma Management Initiatives 1996–99, and will be circulated throughout Scotland for the Scottish Asthma Management Initiative 1998–2001.

CLINICAL ASSESSMENT RECORDING STAMP

Instructions for use: Does the patient answer YES or NO to the following questions?

NO = 0. If YES insert the relevant code number, remember to ask about cough, wheeze, chest tightness or breathlessness.

DATE: Date of clinical assessment		DAYS OFF/LAST MONTH: In the last month has your asthma stopped/severely limited what you would like to do? If so how often? Number of Days:
NIGHT: How many nights in the last month have you had difficulty sleeping because of your asthma symptoms (including cough)? 1 = 1 or 2 x monthly 2 = 1 or 2 x weekly 3 = most nights	DAYTIME: How many days in the last month have you had your usual asthma symptoms during the day (cough, wheeze, chest tightness, or breathlessness)? 1 = 1 or 2 x monthly 2 = 1 or 2 x weekly 3 = daily	ACTIVITY: How many days in the last month has your asthma interfered with your usual activities (eg housework, work/school etc.)? 1 = 1 or 2 x monthly 2 = 1 or 2 x weekly 3 = daily
ACTUAL PEFR: Random measurement at clinical assessment	COMPLIANCE: Satisfactory (S) Unsatisfactory (U)	INHALER TECHNIQUE: Satisfactory (S) Unsatisfactory (U)
% of PREDICTED or BEST:	OTHER EVENTS: RELIEVER MEDICATION: how often has it been used in the last 24 hours	FOLLOW UP: Number of weeks

6. Allen & Hanburys Asthma Audit Instrument

Papers/report

Allen and Hanburys Asthma Audit Instrument (Allen & Hanburys Limited, Uxbridge, Middlesex)

Purpose and setting

A paper-based measuring instrument for use in the patient consultation recorded by nurses. Graphs showing changes in outcome measures produced by Excel spreadsheet.

Description

Nurses running asthma clinics record information collected during the patient consultation on audit record cards (Fig 1) which are kept in the patient notes. The audit record cards are based on the Tayside Asthma Stamp originally developed by the Tayside Asthma Group in Dundee.

Who asks the questions

The audit record cards prompt the nurse to record information on:

- patient symptoms (at night; in the day; on exercise)
- lung function (absolute, or % predicted/best)
- patient compliance with treatment
- inhaler technique
- other events suggestive of poor control (hospitalisations, GP call-outs etc)
- medical interventions suggestive of poor control

Time frame

Night/daytime symptom score:
never; 1–2 per month; 1–2 per week; nightly/daily

Scoring system

Night/day symptom score:
0 = never; 1 = 1–2 per month; 2 = 1–2 per week; 3 = daily/nightly

Activity-induced symptom score:
0 = rarely; 1 = on exercise; 2 = hills/stairs; 3 = walking on flat

Peak expiratory flow:
Record best of three readings (actual), or actual versus predicted/best

Compliance with therapy:
G = good; P = poor

Inhaler technique:
G = good; P = poor

Days off:
Record days off when normal activity restricted.

Interpretation

Nurses are encouraged to audit specific patient groups, eg children, elderly patients, patients with frequent symptoms, and to make treatment and management recommendations in light of the audit results.

The Allen and Hanburys Respiratory Care Team provide a service whereby they process anonymised practice audit data (Fig 2) and generate reports via Excel spreadsheets (Figs 3 and 4) that show changes in the audit measures over the audit period.

Data collected

Use of the audit in over 3,000 practices in the UK has shown significant improvements in patient outcomes. Data on economic outcomes and resource utilisation can also be collected using this measuring instrument (References 1–4 below).

Difficulties have been confronted drawing meaningful conclusions from aggregated data for example, patient cohorts were not matched, and seasonal bias.

However, it has been possible to use this audit instrument to collect and aggregate data at health authority level where specific intention to collect and aggregate data was made clear from the outset.

References

1   Hall JM, Bennett M, Wagg A. The use of fluticasone propionate in the management of severe asthma in a general practice. *Thorax* 1995; **50** (Suppl 2): 6.

2   Price DB, Appleby JL. Fluticasone propionate: an audit of outcomes and cost-effectiveness in primary care. *Respir Med* 1998; **92**: 351–3.

3   Price DB, Cargill K, Wolfe S, Darby H. Salmeterol xinafoate: an analysis of outcomes and cost effectiveness using a primary care database. *Respir Med* 1998; **92**: 1302–4.

4   Ayriss MD, Bruins RH, Davidson M, Goel A, Kaleel MF. Improving asthma care through audit. *Eur Respir J* 1998; **12** (28): 282s.

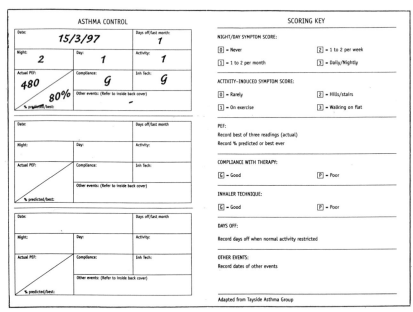

Fig 1. Allen & Hanburys practice asthma audit

Fig 2. Practice audit data

Dr					
Practice Nurse					
Surgery/Health Centre					

Number of patients	48

	START		FINISH	
DATE	05/07/97		04/07/98	

					% Change
NIGHT SYMPTOMS					
Never (0)	26	54%	47	98%	44%
1 to 2 x Monthly (1)	3	6%	1	2%	-4%
1 to 2 x Weekly (2)	3	6%	0	0%	-6%
Daily (3)	16	33%	0	0%	-33%
			Total without symptoms	98%	
			Standard	50%	

DAY SYMPTOMS					
Never (0)	8	17%	40	83%	67%
1 to 2 x Monthly (1)	7	15%	6	13%	-2%
1 to 2 x Weekly (2)	10	21%	0	0%	-21%
Daily (3)	23	48%	2	4%	-44%
			Total without symptoms	83%	
			Standard	50%	

ACTIVITY SYMPTOMS					
Rarely (0)	11	23%	35	73%	50%
On exercise (1)	16	33%	11	23%	-10%
Hills/stairs (2)	13	27%	1	2%	-25%
Walking on Flat (3)	8	17%	0	0%	-17%
			Total without symptoms	73%	
			Standard	40%	

COMPLIANCE					
Good Compliance	43	90%	47	98%	8%
			Good Compliance (G)	98%	
			Standard	90%	

INHALER TECHNIQUE					
Good Inhaler Technique	45	94%	48	100%	6%
			Good Technique (G)	100%	
			Standard	90%	

DAYS OFF (Due to Asthma)					
Patients one or more	7	15%	0	0%	-15%
		Patients who have had one or more day off		0%	
			Standard	50%	

PEAK FLOW					
Total	15400		18100		18%
Average	321		377		
		% Patients whose peak flow improved		85%	
			Standard	50%	

SMOKING		
Yes	0	0%
No	0	0%
Passive	0	0%

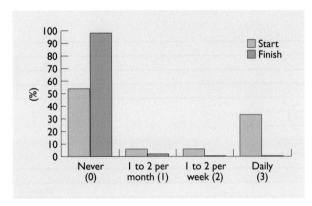

Fig 3. Night-time symptom scores

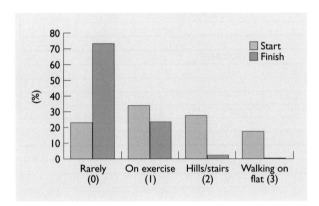

Fig 4. Activity symptom scores

7. Patient indicators in asthma: Integrated Care and Grampian Asthma Practice Study

Papers/reports

1   Drummond N, Abdalla MI, Beattie JB, Buckingham K, Osman LM, Ross S, Russell IT, Douglas JG, Legge JS, Friend JAR. Integrated care: a clinical social and economic evaluation. *Br Med J* 1994; **308**: 559–64.

2   Osman LM, Russell IT, Fiddes J, Friend JAR, Legge JS, Douglas JG. Integrated care for asthma: Matching care to the patient. *Eur Resp J* 1996; **9**: 444–8.

3   Robertson R, Osman LM, Douglas JG. Nurse's role in general practice adult asthma review. *Family Practice* 1997; **14**: 227–32.

Purpose and setting

1)   Integrated Care is a system of shared care for adult asthma patients in Grampian, Scotland. Patients are reviewed annually at chest clinics and seen every 3 months by their GP. At their GP review patients fill in a brief questionnaire on recent symptoms, medication use and asthma control. This information is forwarded to the chest clinic where it is maintained on an ongoing database and reviewed by the patient's consultant.

2)   The Grampian Asthma Practice Study (GAPS) has examined outcomes over 2 years for 1,600 randomly selected adult general practice patients with asthma. Patients were randomly selected for the study from 55 general practices for a 1–4 sample of patients between 16 and 50 years old, who had been prescribed a bronchodilator in the 3 months before the study began.

Description 1 — INTERGRATED CARE

Integrated Care Patient Questionnaire (3-monthly review)

1.	How bad has your asthma been during the last 7 days? *Please tick the answer that describes it best*	
	No wheeze, cough or breathlessness at all	0
	Mild wheeze or cough, not needing any extra treatment	1
	Worsening symptoms needing more treatment than usual, but has not needed you to contact your GP	2
	Severe symptoms needing more treatment and contact with your GP	3
2.	How many courses/booster courses of steroid tablets/injections have you taken in the past 3 months?	[ ] No.
3.	How many times in the past 3 months have you contacted your GP because your asthma has been worse?	[ ] No.
4.	How many times have you visited a hospital emergency department because of asthma in the past 3 months?	[ ] No.
5.	How many times have you been admitted to hospital because of asthma in the past 3 months?	[ ] No.
6.	On how many nights in the past week has your sleep been disturbed by asthma?	[ ] No of nights
7.	Do you have your own peak flow meter?	YES/NO

Who asks the questions

At each 3-monthly review the patient and GP answer two brief questionnaires on recent symptoms, medication use and asthma control.

Integrated care: GP data

```
INTERGRATED CARE
GP Data Collection Questionnaire
(3 months to review)

GP Data Collection

1.  Number of times in the past 3 months
    patient has consulted for troublesome asthma   [ ]

2.  Number of β-agonist relief inhalers patient
    prescribed in the past 9 months                [ ]

3.  Number of corticosteroid inhalers
    prescribed in the past 3 months                [ ]

4.  Number of booster courses of oral steroids
    patient prescribed in the past 3 months.       [ ]


Lung function data
    Date     PEFR (1/min)
             FEV (1/min)
             FVC
```

Data collected

Results on 261 patients

	Per cent of patients in each symptom category having:				
	Two or more bronchodilator scripts	At least one oral steroid course	Any GP acute contact	Any acute hospital attendance (No.)	Mean PEFR
Q1 Asthma control in the past 3 months					
Severe	70%	57%	86%	2	316
Worsening	79%	55%	43%	0	327
Mild	68%	27%	35%	3	336
No symptoms	50%	11%	14%	2	405
p	<0.05	<0.01	<0.001		<0.01
Q6 Sleep disturbance week before review					
Every night	71%	57%	57%	0	301
4–6 nights	100%	56%	67%	0	272
1–3 nights	70%	46%	54%	3	332
no nights	65%	23%	29%	4	354
p	NS	<0.01	<0.001		NS

Data collected

Results on 357 patients

Asthma control 3 months before review	Severe, needing GP contact	6%
	Worsening, but not needing GP contact	14%
	Mild wheeze, no extra treatment	61%
	No wheeze/breathlessness	18%
Sleep disturbance week before review	Every night	3%
	4–6 nights	4%
	1–3 nights	23%
	No disturbed nights in past week	70%

Asthma control was significantly linearly related (p<0.001) to:
- number of oral steroid courses in previous 3 months
- number of GP acute visits in previous 3 months
- PEFR

Sleep disturbance was significantly linearly related (p<0.001) to
- number of oral steroid courses in previous 3 months
- it was less strongly, and not linearly related to GP contact
- it was not related to PEFR

Asthma control was non linearly related (p<0.01) to bronchodilator prescriptions, ie the difference was between those with no symptoms vs any level of symptoms.

Sleep disturbance was not related to bronchodilator prescriptions.

Description 2 — GAPS (GRAMPIAN ASTHMA PRACTICE STUDY)

GAPS Patient Questionnaire
(1 month before interview)

In the past month how often have you been wheezy or breathless during the day?

Every day
At least one day every week
Occasionally, not every week
Not at all

In the past month how often has cough or breathlessness disturbed your sleep?

Every day
At least one day every week
Occasionally, not every week
Not at all

In the past year how many bad attacks of asthma have you had?

None 1 2 3 4 5

GAPS GP Data Collection Questionnaire
(12 months before interview)

GP Data Collection (from Note Review)

1. Number of times in the past 12 months patient has consulted for troublesome asthma [ ]

2. Number of β-agonist relief inhalers patient prescribed in the past 12 months [ ]

3. Number of corticosteroid inhalers prescribed in the past 12 months [ ]

4. Number of booster courses of oral steroids patient prescribed in the past 12 months. [ ]

Home interview. Lung function data
Date   PEFR (1/min)
            FEV (1/min)
            FVC

Home interview:
SF36
St George's Respiratory Questionnaire
Hospital Anxiety and Depression Questionnaire

GAPS patient questionnaire	Association with quality-of-life measures		Eta ‡
Q1 Day wheeze in the past month	St. George's Respiratory Q:	Symptoms	0.54 *
		Impact	0.46 *
		Activity	0.43 *
	SF-12 Generic:	Physical (6 Qs)	0.40 *
		Mental (6 Qs)	0.20 †
	HADS:	Anxiety	0.19 *
		Depression	0.16 †
Q2 Sleep disturbance in the past month	St. George's Respiratory Q:	Symptoms	0.54 *
		Impact	0.51 *
		Activity	0.38 *
	SF-12:	Physical (6 Qs)	0.35 *
		Mental (6 Qs)	0.16 †
	HADS:	Anxiety	0.16 †
		Depression	0.21 *
Q3 Attacks in past 12 months (Patient report)	St. George's Respiratory Q:	Symptoms	0.56 *
		Impact	0.45 *
		Activity	0.44 *
	SF-12:	Physical (6 Qs)	0.39 *
		Mental (6 Qs)	0.21 *
	HADS:	Anxiety	0.19 *
		Depression	0.24 *

* $p < 0.001$ † $p < 0.01$ ‡ Eta correlation coefficient, varies between -1 and +1

Interpretation

Integrated Care

▌ There was not a linear relationship between bronchodilator prescriptions and symptoms. Patients with moderate symptoms were almost as likely to use high numbers of bronchodilators as those with severe symptoms of breathlessness. Only patients who reported no symptoms used bronchodilators significantly less.

▌ The clinical indicator best related to asthma control was GP acute contact in the past 3 months. The indicator best related to sleep disturbance was number of steroid courses used in the past 3 months.

Grampian Asthma Practice Study

▌ The GAPS patients are a milder group of asthmatics than Integrated Care patients. They are younger and have better lung function.

▌ All patients in Integrated Care have been referred to specialist care, but only 19% of GAPS patients have been in specialist care in the past 10 years.

▌ GAPS patients used fewer bronchodilator prescriptions, took fewer steroid courses and made fewer acute GP visits. Nonetheless, as for Integrated Care, steroid courses and acute GP visits are significantly related to day wheeze and night disturbance in the past month, and attacks in the past year, as was found for the more severe Integrated Care group.

Quality of life and patient symptom report

▌ Simple symptom questions relate to clinical indicator both for community populations and clinic populations of asthmatics.

▌ Relationships of current reported symptoms with acute visits and steroid courses are found in the short term (3 months) and longer term (12 months).

▋ SF 12 generic quality-of-life questions, referring to health status in the past month, are powerfully related to symptom questions for that month in a community population, and relate to GP acute visits and oral steroid courses over 12 months.

▋ Choice of outcome indicators will depend on what clinicians and patients want to change.

8. Ambulatory Care Asthma Measure
(Department of Public Health Medicine, University of Hull)

Papers

1   Steen N, Hutchinson A, McColl E, Eccles MP, Hewison J, Meadows KA, Blades SM, Fowler P. Development of a symptom based outcome measure for asthma. *Br Med J* 1994; **309**: 1065–8.

2   McColl E, Steen N, Meadows KA, Hutchinson A, Eccles MP, Hewison J, Fowler P, Blades SM. Developing outcome measures for ambulatory care: an application to asthma and diabetes. *Soc Sci Med* 1995; **41**: 1339–48.

Purpose and setting

- Need for condition-specific, patient-centred outcome measures.

- As **an outcome indicator**: a measure of health used quantitatively to describe the health of a group of people in a specific setting.

- As **an outcome assessment measure**: used over time to attribute observed changes to a particular intervention, such as introduction of structured care; describing the impact of care; providing information for reliable decision making, such as in medical audit; and evaluating the effectiveness of care in defined circumstances.

- Applicable in an ambulatory setting (general practice and hospital outpatients).

Description

A practical, condition-specific measurement tool for adults that is patient-centred, multi-domain, outcome and effectiveness oriented.

Who asks the questions

The questionnaire is self completed. It is currently being used in routine evaluation of health care by the authors and others in a number of ongoing programmes.

Time frame

It was necessary to strike a balance between a time frame that was too long, perhaps leading to a recall bias, and too short, which might lead to low item endorsement. One month was chosen as a recall period for items asking about symptom frequency and 3 months for items asking about more memorable events such as time off work and consultations with doctors.

Scoring system

A five-point scale was used for all 10 questions, ranging from 'never' to 'every day' because it was felt unreasonable to expect the patient to recall the exact number of days on which symptoms had been experienced. Individual question responses are scored from 1 to 4, the results aggregated and transformed to obtain a single value.

Interpretation

Testing the questionnaire. The questionnaire was piloted on groups of patients to ensure that each item could be easily understood. It was also tested for internal reliability, test-retest reliability, and endorsement of response categories (see Tables 1–4).

The questionnaire is designed as a population measure and is not suitable for interpretation on an individual level. The work towards developing a symptom-based outcome measure for asthma showed that condition-specific measures may be more responsive to change than generic measures.

Data collected

AMBULATORY CARE ASTHMA MEASURE

___

Asthma symptoms — about these questions

These questions are about your asthma. They ask about your symptoms over the past month.

To answer the questions, **please circle the number** that **best** describes how you have been over the past month.

Each question describes a possible symptom of asthma and asks you to say **how often** in the **past month** you have felt like that.

For each question please **circle the number** that best describes how you have been in the past month. Make sure that you circle only one number for each question.

___

C1　In the **past month**, on how many **days** have you been short of breath **during exercise?**
　　(for example, going upstairs, walking uphill, gardening, taking part in sports)

never	on one or a few days	on several days	on most days	every day
1	2	3	4	5

___

C2　In the **past month**, on how many **days** have you been short of breath **during the day** at times when **you were not exercising?**

Never	on one or a few days	on several days	on most days	every day
1	2	3	4	5

___

C3　In the past month, on how many days have you wheezed during the day?

Never	on one or a few days	on several days	on most days	every day
1	2	3	4	5

___

C4　In the **past month**, on how many **days** have you coughed **during the day?**

Never	on one or a few days	on several days	on most days	every day
1	2	3	4	5

___

C5　In the **past month**, on how many **nights** have you wheezed?

Never	on one or a few days	on several days	on most days	every day
1	2	3	4	5

___

C6　In the **past month**, on how many **nights** have you been short of breath?

Never	on one or a few days	on several days	on most days	every day
1	2	3	4	5

___

C7　In the **past month**, on how many **nights** have you coughed?

Never	on one or a few days	on several days	on most days	every day
1	2	3	4	5

___

C8　In the **past month**, on how many **nights** have you had problems sleeping because of a cough or chest problems (for example, bother getting to sleep or being woken in the night)?

Never	on one or a few days	on several days	on most days	every day
1	2	3	4	5

___

C9　In the **past month**, on how many **days** have you felt frightened because of your asthma?

Never	on one or a few days	on several days	on most days	every day
1	2	3	4	5

___

C10　In the **past month**, on how many **days** has your chest felt tight?

Never	on one or a few days	on several days	on most days	every day
1	2	3	4	5

___

Table 1. Concurrent and predictive validity of the 10-item asthma symptom questionnaire; values are Spearman rank-order correlation coefficients (Table from Steen *et al*, reference 1 above. *Reproduced by permission of BMJ*)

Symptom score	Symptom level		Doctors' evaluation of 10-item asthma	
Criteria	Concurrent validity *	Predictive validity †	Concurrent validity *	Predictive validity †
Number of asthma attacks	0.45	0.44	0.32	0.27
Chest infections	0.47	0.37	0.36	0.30
Routine consultations	0.53	0.57	0.37	0.42
Unplanned consultations	0.36	0.53	0.35	0.26
Impaired activity	0.56	0.53	0.34	0.34

* Scale scores were correlated with the adverse occurrences (the criteria) which occurred during the 3 months before the questionnaire.
† In assessing predictive validity, scale scores were correlated with the adverse occurrences which occurred in the 3 months after the questionnaire.

Table 2. Coefficients (99% confidence intervals) for correlation of alternative forms of asthma symptom score with criterion index (From Steen *et al*, 1 above. *Reproduced by permission of BMJ*)

Scale	Concurrent validity Correlation coefficient (99% confidence interval)	Predictive validity Correlation coefficient (99% confidence interval)
Total symptom score	0.68 (0.62 to 0.74)	0.59 (0.48 to 0.69)
Weighted symptom score	0.68 (0.62 to 0.74)	0.58 (0.47 to 0.68)
Reduced scale 1	0.65 (0.59 to 0.71)	0.58 (0.46 to 0.68)
Reduced scale 2	0.66 (0.59 to 0.72)	0.57 (0.45 to 0.67)
SF-36 general health perception scale	0.58 (0.46 to 0.68)	0.53 (0.33 to 0.68)

Table 3. Change in asthma symptom score by patients' perception of change in their asthma. (From Steen *et al*, 1 above. *Reproduced by permission of BMJ*)

Perception of change	Mean change (95% confidence interval)
Much better (n=26)	⁻15.0 (⁻23.1 to ⁻6.9)
A little better (n=36)	6.0 (⁻11.1 to 0.9)
About the same (n=142)	⁻0.4 (2.9 to 2.2)
A little worse (n=40)	5.2 (⁻0.4 to 10.8)
Much worse (n=5)	⁻1.0 (⁻14.5 to 12.6)

Table 4. Change in total symptom score for 26 patients reporting much improvement in their asthma (From Steen *et al*, 1 above. *Reproduced by permission of BMJ*))

Scale	Mean score		τ- Value	p- value	Effect size
	Baseline	Follow-up			
Total symptom score	14.5	8.5	3.65	<0.001	0.66
Weighted symptom score	14.9	9.7	3.78	<0.001	0.70
Reduced scale 1	8.1	4.9	3.85	<0.001	0.65
Reduced scale 2	8.1	4.7	3.57	<0.001	0.64
SF-36 general health perception scale *	58.9	55.8	−0.79†	0.72†	−0.14

* The SF-36 is scaled such that an increase in the score represents an improvement in health status
† The SF-36 was administered to a subset of patients only; calculations are based on 13 cases

9. Northampton Asthma Survey

Papers/reports

1   Jeffrey M, Meadows K, Greene T and Jeffrey AA. Northampton Asthma Survey: results of a postal questionnaire. *Thorax* 1996; **51**: 62.

Purpose and setting

The Northampton Asthma Project was set up to establish a means by which those involved in asthma care could collaborate and gain information about the health of people with asthma living in and around Northampton. The project used the questionnaire devised by the Department of Public Health Medicine at the University of Hull along with an abbreviated Hospital Anxiety and Depression score, an assessment of physical function and energy levels.

The aims of the survey were:

- to quantify morbidity in adults diagnosed as having asthma and living in our community
- to explore links between asthma morbidity and the provision and use of local health services

Description

The questionnaire included the following items:

- asthma symptoms
- anxiety and depression indices
- physical activity
- energy levels
- prescription and use of inhaled steroids and peak flow meters
- emergency and routine medical attendance

COMPONENTS OF ASTHMA SYMPTOM SCORE

In the last month:

- How many days were you short of breath during exercise?
- How many days were you short of breath while not exercising?
- How many days have you wheezed during the day?
- How many days have you coughed during the day?
- How many nights have you wheezed?
- How many nights were you short of breath?
- How many nights did you cough?
- How many nights have you had difficulty sleeping because of cough or chest problems?
- How many days have you been frightened because of your asthma?
- How many days has your chest felt tight?

Who asks the questions

Postal questionnaire with one reminder, if no response, in 2 weeks.

Practice selection: all practices invited to take part (approximately 1 in 3 agreed).

Patient selection:

- Age 18–60 years inclusive
- Diagnosis of asthma recorded by general practitioner
- Minimum of one prescription for a bronchodilator in the last 12 months
- Random selection from complete list of eligible patients
- Sample size of 1% of practice list for each practice

Time Frame

One month

Scoring system:

Five-point scale for asthma symptoms using the Steen *et al* ambulatory care asthma measure in a postal setting without any apparent loss in usefulness.

Never	One or a few days	On several days	On most days	Every day
1	2	3	4	5

The score is calculated as a composite of the ten responses and has a range of 0 to 100. The wide range of possible responses is potentially useful in making comparisons with other graded outcome measures.

Interpretation

- The random sample of adults with asthma represents approximately 1 in 5 of the adults in the practices surveyed (assuming a prevalence of asthma of 5% of adults)
- There is a significant association between asthma symptoms and other health measures with potential impairment of life quality. The Asthma Symptom Score may be useful as an outcome measure.
- A high asthma symptom score is associated with current or previous regular smoking.
- Patients with high asthma symptom scores are more likely to require emergency consultations, but the spread of results limits the usefulness of the score in predicting individual needs.
- Patients admitting to not taking prescribed preventive medication do not seem to suffer worse symptoms than those who claim to take it.
- Differences in patterns of care between practices are not shown to influence overall symptoms.
- Daytime chest tightness has also been compared with other responses to do with daytime symptoms. The data demonstrate individual variability but when aggregated the differences do not appear major.

Data collected

Response

1,176 questionnaires were issued; 706 analysable responses were received (response rate = 60%)

Patient demographics

Sex	Male 45%	Female 55%
Mean age	Male 37.6 years	Female 37.8 years
Asthma symptom score (mean)	Male 30.7	Female 34.3 ($p=0.03$)

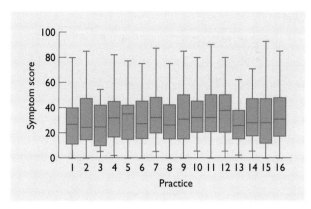

Fig 1. Asthma symptom score by practice

There was no significant difference in overall asthma symptom scores between any of the 16 practices taking part in this study (Fig. 1). This uniformity of asthma symptoms was found despite the differences between practices in the organisation of their asthma care and patterns of received care in the patients sampled from each practice.

To put the score in some context, the bar chart in Fig. 2 shows the response to the item on night-time symptoms. In this sample, there was a mean score of 30.7 (male) and 34.3 (female); 14.4% of respondents were disturbed most or every night.

There was significant correlation between the Asthma Symptom Score and other indicators of general health, in this case the depression component of the abbreviated HAD (Hospital Anxiety Depression). The correlation line and its 95% confidence intervals are shown in Fig.3.

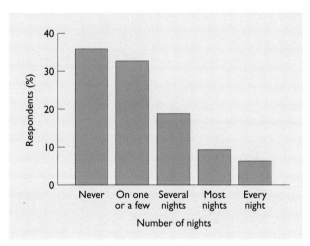

Fig 2. Sleep disturbed by cough or chest problems in past month

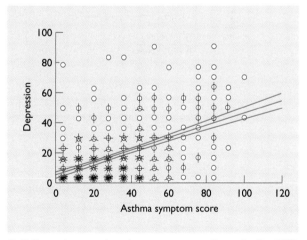

Fig 3. Depression score by asthma symptom score. Regression line +95% CI (r = 0.49)

10. Blackpool Asthma Care Plan

Papers/report

O'Reilly JF, Berry P. *Blackpool Asthma Care Plan.* Blackpool Victoria Hospital NHS Trust.

Purpose and setting

A patient-centred system for the management and education of patients with asthma throughout the Blackpool district. The system is tailored to individual patient needs in education, monitoring and drug therapy. The aims of the system include:

- annual audit
- anonymity
- audit reports to GP practices

Description

During the past 3 months	Appt./Date
Symptoms average days/weeks: Cough, Sputum, Tightness, Breathlessness, Wheeze 3 Daily, 2 Weekly, I Occasional Nights woken by symptoms I/52 Best peak flow Worst peak flow Inhaler device Inhaler technique corrected (yes/no) Acute GP visits Days off work/school Oral steroid courses Reliever average dose/day	

Who asks the questions

The patient-held record and advice card allows shared care between the patient, general practice, and hospital asthma clinic.

Time frame

During the past 3 months.

Scoring system

Asthma symptoms: daily = 3; weekly = 2; occasionally = 1

Nights woken by symptoms per week:

Days off work: number over 3/12

Interpretation

Cross-sectional measurement of severity. Measures symptoms (1 week); nights woken (1 week); days off work/ school (3 months); visits to GP (3 months); steroid courses (3 months); reliever use per day; step of treatment.

Longitudinal measure of change. Card provides a record of change and audit repeated individually by visit and annually across the practice.

Predictive outcome. Asthma plan includes Jones morbidity index predictors: nocturnal wheeze; time off work; wheezy symptoms.

Data collected

Pilot study; 3-man practice; 8,000 population; 418 on the Asthma Register; 308 on the Asthma Plan Card

Comparison of level of control with steps of treatment allows precise individual management

PRACTICE A

Symptoms	Nights woken	Days off work
65% completed	56% completed	40.6% completed
40% without symptoms	49% no wakening	39% no days off
25% with symptoms	7% wakening	1.6% with days off
35% incomplete	44% incomplete	59.4% incomplete
17% ambiguous	2% ambiguous	

Steroid courses	Acute gp visits	Steps of treatment	
43% completed	43.5% completed	Step 1	11%
40% no course required	38% no visits	Step 2	59%
3% course required	5.5% acute visits	Step 3	19%
		Step 4	8%
57% incomplete	56.5% incomplete	Step 5	3%

Conclusions

- Asthma Card is viable and widely used (34 practices involved)
- More information is collected than previously available. (Appendix A, Figs 1 and 2)
- Data value is compromised if incomplete
- Ambiguity of symptom criteria even when 96.4% complete. (Appendix A, Figs 3 and 4)
- Entries often descriptive rather than quantitative

Strategy for change:
- Refine criteria and remove ambiguity
- Promote accurate card completion
- Encourage categorisation rather than description
- Add assessment of exercise capacity
- Add patient goal
- Validate revised card

Appendix A. Asthma Care Plan record card

During the past month:	eg Date 15/07/98												
Have you had your usual asthma symptoms during the day? Y/N	Y												
If YES daily = 3 weekly = 2 occas = 1	3												
Have you had difficulty sleeping because of your asthma symptoms (including cough)?Y/N	Y												
If YES daily = 3 weekly = 2 occas = 1	2												
Since last visit													
Has your asthma interfered with your usual activities (eg housework/work/school)? Y/N	Y												
If YES number of days since last visit	4												
Number of acute visits	1												
H = Hospital G = G.P. N = Nurse	G												
Oral steroid courses	0												
Number of hospital admissions	0												
Best peak flow	400												
Today's peak flow	300												
Height if applicable	N/A												
Inhaler technique, Good? Y/N	Y												

Treatments: Drug name (If puffs per day less than one write <1)	device/ tablet	dose per puff	puffs per day	device/ tablet	dose per puff	puffs per day	device/ tablet	dose per puff	puffs per day	device/ tablet	dose per puff	puffs per day
STEP 1: TERBUTALINE	T	500 mcg	6									
STEP 2: BUDESONIDE	MS	200 mcg	4									
STEP 3: SALMETEROL	A	50 mcg	2									
STEP 4: OXITROPIUM	MS	100 mcg	4									
STEP 5:												

Device: M (M.D.I) **S** (SPACER) **AUTO** (AUTOHALER) **E** (EASYBREATHE) **A** (ACCUHALER) **D** (DISKHALER) **T** (TURBOHALER) **P** (POWDER) **O** (ORAL)

Advice: also see peak flow diary	patient has increased budesonide, morning dip persists & nightime wakening add salmeterol b.d				
PATIENT GOAL	To go swimming & sleep without the need for a reliever				
ACHIEVED Y/N	N				

Fig 1. Symptoms recording from various sources — Practice A

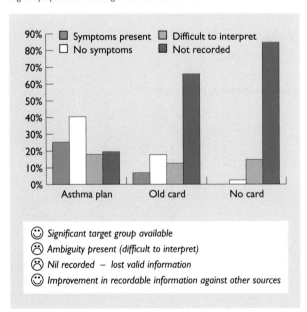

☺ Significant target group available
☹ Ambiguity present (difficult to interpret)
☹ Nil recorded — lost valid information
☺ Improvement in recordable information against other sources

Fig 2. Night-time wakening from various sources — Practice A

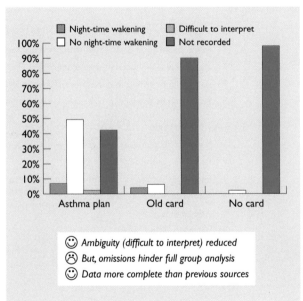

☺ Ambiguity (difficult to interpret) reduced
☹ But, omissions hinder full group analysis
☺ Data more complete than previous sources

Fig 3. Comparison of symptom recording between two practices —
Asthma plan only

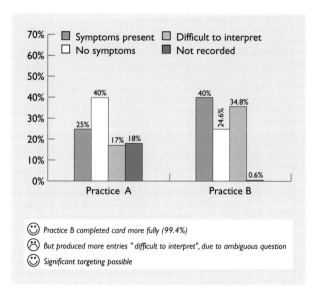

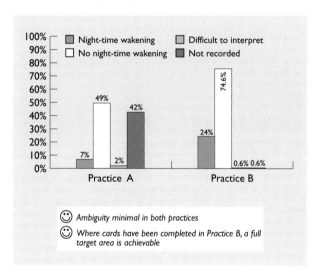

Fig 4. Comparison of night-time wakening recording between two
practices — Asthma plan only

11. Salford Asthma Register

Papers/report

1   Ansted SJ, MacDowell D, O'Driscoll BR (On behalf of START). The Salford Asthma Register: a mechanism for auditing a district asthma population and supporting GP asthma care (Abstract). *Thorax* 1998; **53**: A75.

Purpose and setting

The Salford Asthma Register was launched at the beginning of 1995. It aims to provide an IT system for the registration, annual review and feedback of data to general practices on the status of their registered asthmatic patients.

The Salford & Trafford Asthma and Respiratory Team (START) developed the minimum data set and encouraged every general practice in Salford to collect data as a means of standardising the quality of care.

Description

▌   Asthma status

▌   Previous reviews

▌   Clinical review

▌   Quality of life

Who asks the questions

Once a year the general practitioner or practice nurse completes a review sheet for each active asthma patient who attends a clinic.

Time frame

Day and night symptoms

Day and night asthma symptoms are recorded according to the whole period since the last registration.

The register asks if nocturnal symptoms occur nightly, weekly or monthly.

Quality of life

Time off work or school as a consequence of asthma is asked for the last month.

How much has asthma been interfering with your life over the last year?

Are you happy with the asthma care you have received over the last year?

Scoring System

Day time symptoms   0 = no symptoms;   1 = symptoms running;   2 = symptoms climbing stairs; 3 = symptoms walking on flat;   4 = symptoms at rest.

Nocturnal symptoms: 0 = none;   1 = one or two episodes of wakening per month; 2 = one or two episodes of wakening per week;   3 = one or more episodes every night.

Interpretation

▌   It is possible to establish a district asthma database that covers the majority of known asthma patients

▌   Such a database can provide useful GP feedback reports and important asthma audit data

▌   A district can use these data to identify areas of strength and areas for improvement in asthma management.

Data collected

RESULTS

▌ 10,837 asthmatics registered from 41 general practices covering over 70% of the Salford population.

▌ 2,086 (19.2%) of the asthmatics have had an annual review and 1,470 (13.6%) have been recorded as resolved.

▌ 1,009 (56.7%) patients are in British Thoracic Society (BTS) category 2 — low-dose inhaled steroid or cromoglycate (see Fig. 1).

▌ 276 (13.5%) patients reviewed suffer from nightly symptoms (Fig. 2), with 53.3% (147) of these are in BTS category 1 or 2.

▌ 552 (28.6%) patients have had at least one GP-treated exacerbation in the last 12 months, with 53.3% (294) of these in BTS category 1 or 2 (Fig 4).

▌ 852 (41.8%) asthmatics in Salford have no daytime symptoms.

▌ 42.8% (521) of those reviewed have their own self-management plan.

▌ PEFR as percent predicted was found to be lower in BTS category 1 than in category 2 (Fig. 4).

All 41 practices received reports providing them with a printout of their data compared to the districts.

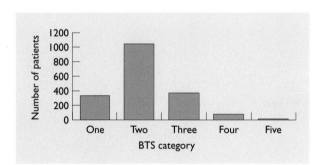

Fig 1. BTS Category. Number of patients with their BTS category recorded = 1,781 (85.4%)

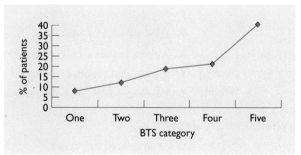

Fig 3. BTS vs Nightly symptoms. Number of patients who are suffering nightly symptoms = 276 (13.5%)

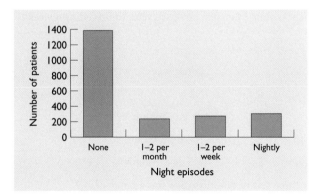

Fig 2. Night symptoms. Number of patients with night symptoms recorded = 2,039 (97.7%)

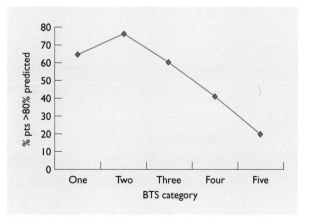

Fig 4. Predicted PEFR vs BTS category. Number of patients with data recorded = 821 (39.4%)

12. Norwich Asthma Control Study

Papers/reports:

1 Harrison BDW, Kelly Y, Sodergren S Wilkes A, Hyland M, Watkin SW. Attempts to assess asthma control in a hospital outpatient population. *Thorax* 1998; **53**: A75.

Purpose and setting

To evaluate different measures of asthma control in a routine respiratory clinic setting. Data were collected from newly referred asthmatics attending the Norfolk and Norwich Hospital respiratory medicine outpatients clinic.

Description

- Hyland Living with Asthma Questionnare (LWAQ)
- Norwich Asthma Questionnaire
- Norwich Asthma Management Card

The Norwich Asthma Questionnaire and Management Card cover:

- Admissions to hospital
- Unscheduled contacts with doctor or nurse
- Nights disturbed by asthma
- Days off work or education
- Asthma bother socially, domestically or personally
- Prednisolone courses or boosts
- Days when PEF falls below 80% and 60% best

Who asks the questions

- LWAQ completed by patient
- Norwich Asthma Questionnaire completed by patient and doctor
- Norwich Asthma Management Card completed by patient and data abstracted by doctor

Time frame

Both the Norwich Asthma Questionnaire and Norwich Asthma Management Card refer to preceding 4 weeks.

Scoring system

Sleep		Work/study		Other ways	
No =	0	No =	0	No =	0
<once/week =	1	<1 day/month =	1	<1 day/month =	1
1–4 nights/week =	2	1–4 days/month =	2	1–4 days/month =	2
≥ 5 nights/week =	3	≥5 days/month =	3	≥5 days/month =	3

Total asthma score is the sum of the answers to these three sets of questions and has a range of 0–9.

Interpretation

- Missing values in a study conducted in a busy clinic by interested physicians emphasise the importance of developing 'user friendly' indices of control of asthma which will be employed in such a setting.
- Asthma quality of life, symptom scores, peak flows at home and lung function in the clinic all showed improvement following referral to the clinic (Tables 1–4)

- Associated with this improvement patients were regularly receiving more treatment and were less often requiring to step their treatment up. They were also taking less prednisolone. (Table 3).

- There was good correlation between the symptom of sleep disturbance due to asthma recorded on the Management Card and recalled at the clinic visit (Table 5).

- PEF falling below 80% best in the preceding month correlated poorly with disturbance at work, study or other activities, better but not significantly with sleep disturbance ($p=0.072$) and best with total asthma score ($p=0.04$) (Table 6).

- Interval clinic PEF and FEV_1 correlated very well with whether or not PEF at home fell below 80% best in the previous week or month and whether or not the patient had taken or boosted their prednisolone (Table 7).

- Changes in clinic PEF but not FEV_1 correlated with disturbances of work, study or other activities but not with sleep disturbance (Table 8).

The Norwich Asthma Control Study are grateful to Glaxo-Wellcome UK for a non- promotional grant in support of this study and to Mrs Alison Neale for her expertise and help in documentation and presentation.

Table 1. Mean (range) LWAQ total and construct scores (n=9)

	Baseline	2 months	6 months
Total	0.87 (0.22–1.18)	0.74 (0.19–1.21)	0.75 (0.04–1.17)
Avoidance	0.81 (0.39–1.06)	0.63 (0.24–1.33)	0.77 (0.00–1.44)
Preoccupation	1.04 (0.40–1.60)	1.10 (0.30–1.80)	0.78 (0.11–1.50)
Activities	0.82 (0.60–1.33)	0.73 (0.63–1.44)	0.72 (0.00–1.50)
Distress	0.86 (0.16–1.59)	0.63 (0.05–1.24)	0.70 (0.05–1.24)

Note: 0 = very good quality of life, 2 = very poor quality of life

Table 2. Results from the Norwich Asthma Questionnaire (n=12) — all in previous 4 weeks

	Baseline	2 months	6 months
No sleep disturbance	2	2	6
Woken >1 night/week	6	1	2
No asthma bother at work/study	4	3	6
No asthma bother socially, domestically, personally	5	3	7
No prednisolone courses or boosts	8	10	12

Table 3. Mean (range) values for items on the Norwich Asthma Management Card (n=13) — all in the previous month

	Baseline	2 months	6 months
Emergency consultations	0.5 (0–2)	0.15 (0.2)	0.08 (0–1)
Days off work/school	2.7 (0–7)	1.33 (0–14)	0 (0)
Nights disturbed	7.0 (0–24)	2.17 (0–10)	2.15 (0–12)
Usual treatment step	3.0 (1–5)	3.58 (3–4)	3.92 (3–5)
Treatment step increased	2.4 (0–10)	0.54 (0–7)	1.0 (0–7)
Days prednisolone taken	5.55 (0–30)	3.23 (0–30)	3.23 (0–30)
Days peak flow <80% best	14.2 (0–28)	12.3 (0–27)	7.42 (0–28)
Days peak flow <60% best	2.9 (0-13)	0.55 (0-4)	0.15 (0-2)
PEF as % predicted	76.4 (48-95)	107.9 (106-111)	84.5 (82-87)
FEV_1 as % predicted	77.6 (39-98)	95.6 (88-108)	81.2 (66-96)
Best PEF at home	416 (250-520)	445 (300-640)	440 (320-640)

Table 4. Comparison of clinic lung function and total asthma score at first and last visit — mean (SD)

	First visit	Last visit	p
PEF (1/min) $\Big\}$ N=17	354 (87.8)	375 (81.5)	0.13
FEV$_1$ (1)	2.44 (0.71)	2.61 (0.8)	0. 054
Asthma score n=15	4.33 (3.38)	2.0 (2.81)	0.065

Table 5. Agreement between answers to questions from two sources (Norwich Asthma Questionnaire and Management Card) about waking from sleep due to asthma in the week before clinic visit

	Norwich Asthma Questionnaire	
Management Card	No (N=34)	Yes (N=19)
No (n=24)	24	0
Yes (n=29)	10	19

Therefore, for 43 (19+24) of 53 visits there was agreement between the answers given to the questions about waking from sleep due to asthma.

Pearson chi square = 24.5   Significance, p = 0.0001

Table 6. In the previous month

	Waking from sleep		Work/study disturbance		Other activities disturbance		Total asthma score		
PEF <80% best in preceding month	no	yes	no	yes	no	yes	0	1–4	5–9
No	13	8	17	5	17	4	13	6	3
Yes	8	15	14	8	15	8	7	8	8
χ^2	3.24		0.98		1.37		5.726		
p	0.072		0.32		0.24		0.04		

Table 7. Clinic lung function — mean (SD) — compared with:

whether PEF fell below 80% best in the previous week

	No (n=32)	Yes (n=23)	p
% predicted PEF	96.9 (14.4)	72.6 (18.7)	0.0001
% predicted FEV$_1$	99.8 (14.3)	68.2 (20.2)	0.0001

number of days PEF fell below 80% best in the previous month

	0 (23 patients)	1–7 (13 patients)	8–28 (16 patients)	p
% predicted PEF	92.7 (16.2)	95.7 (17.7)	69.8 (19)	0.0001
% predicted FEV$_1$	99 (16.8)	91 (20.8)	65.8 (20.3)	0.0001

whether patient had taken prednisolone or boosted the dose in the previous month

	No (n=28)	Yes (n=10)	p
% predicted PEF	95.8 (17.8)	74.7 (15.7)	0.004
% predicted FEV$_1$	98.2 (17.1)	72.4 (20.6)	0.0001

Table 8. Changes in lung function — mean (SD) — compared with patients' perception of how asthma affects them symptomatically, at that visit compared with first attendance at clinic

Sleep Disturbance (n=55)

	Same (n=5)	Improved (n=21)	Very much better (n=29)	p
Change in PEF (1/min)	3.0 (46.7)	17.2 (50.8)	30.0 (48.9)	0.44
Change in FEV$_1$	⁻0.016 (0.33)	0.148 (0.22)	0.246 (0.34)	0.17

Work / Study Disturbance (n=53)

	Same (n=12)	Improved (n=12)	Very much better (n=29)	p
Change in PEF (1/min)	⁻1.25 (56.4)	6.9 (28)	39.1 (48.6)	0.022
Change In FEV$_1$	0.08 (0.31)	0.178 (0.23)	0.23 (0.33)	0.37

Social, Domestic, Personal Disturbance (n=55)

	Same (n=17)	Improved (n=17)	Very much better (n=21)	p
Change in PEF (1/min)	9.7 (56.1)	7.3 (35.4)	44 (46)	0.034
Change in FEV$_1$	0.08 (0.29)	0.184 (0.21)	0.268 (0.35)	0.17

Data collected

NORWICH ASTHMA QUESTIONNAIRE [FOLLOW-UP VISIT]

How many times have you been admitted to hospital with your asthma in the last WEEK; MONTH; 3 MONTHS; 6 MONTHS; YEAR

None	0
Once	1
Twice	2
3 times	3
4 times	4
More than 4 times	5

How many times have you visited your doctor or practice nurse, called your doctor out or visited the accident and emergency department for unscheduled appointments and urgent treatment of your asthma in the last WEEK; MONTH; 3 MONTHS; 6 MONTHS; YEAR

None	0
Once	1
Twice	2
3 times	3
4 times	4
More than 4 times	5

continued opposite

Compared to how you were before coming to the clinic, has your asthma been better or worse during the night?

(Please tick one) Very much better

Better

Slightly better

Just noticeably better

No difference

Just noticeably worse

Slightly worse

Very much worse

Has it woken you from sleep in the last 4 weeks?

No	0
< once/week	1
1–4 nights/week	2
> 5 nights/week	3
Several times each night	4

Compared to how you were before coming to the clinic, has there been any changes in the way asthma has bothered you at work or study?

(Please tick one) Very much better

Better

Slightly better

Just noticeably better

No difference

Just noticeably worse

Slightly worse

Very much worse

Has it bothered you at work or study in the last 4 weeks?

No	0
<1 day/month	1
1–4 days/month	2
5–10 days/month	3
> 10 days/month	4

Compared to how you were before coming to the clinic, has there been any change in the way asthma has bothered you in any other way (for example, social activities, domestic activities, personal activities)

(Please tick one) Very much better

Better

Slightly better

Just noticeably better

No difference

Just noticeably worse

Slightly worse

Very much worse

Has it bothered you in these other ways in the last 4 weeks?

No	0
<1 day/month	1
1–4 days/month	2
5–10 days/month	3
> 10 days/month	4

Do you take prednisolone (steroid) tablets for your asthma?

No

Yes   If yes   .... every day?   .... short courses?

**Have you had to increase ('boost') your daily dose of prednisolone
or start a short course in the last WEEK; MONTH; 3 MONTHS; 6 MONTHS;YEAR**

None	0
Once	1
Twice	2
More than twice	3

13. Greenwich Asthma Study: Evaluation of a community intervention trial on the management of asthma

Papers/reports

1 Marks GB, Burney PG, Premaratne UN, Simpson J and Webb J. Asthma in Greenwich, UK: impact of the disease and current management practices. *Eur Resp J* 1997; **6**: 1224–9. (Gives study design and baseline data)

2 Premaratne UN, Sterne JAC, Marks GB, Webb JR, Azima H and Burney PGJ. Clustered randomised trial of an intervention to improve the management of asthma: Greenwich Asthma Study. *Br Med J* 1999; **318**: 1251–55.

Purpose and setting

To evaluate the effectiveness of an Asthma Resource Centre (ARC) in improving treatment and quality of life for patients with asthma through community-wide implementation of the British Thoracic Society's guidelines.

Community-randomised trial, among 41 general practices in Greenwich that had a practice nurse responsible for running asthma clinics. In general practices in which the intervention was carried out, asthma nurse specialists educated and supported practice nurses, who in turn educated patients on the management of asthma according to British Thoracic Society guidelines. The trial was evaluated using two surveys (in 1994 and 1997) each of 24,000 patients aged 15–50 years and registered with the general practices. The effect of the intervention on attendance at local A&E departments for asthma, and prescribing of asthma medication, was also evaluated.

Description

Screening questionnaire, with longer questionnaire, including an asthma quality of life questionnaire (AQLQ) for patients defined as asthmatic, and other questions on asthma severity and treatment.

GREENWICH RESPIRATORY HEALTH SURVEY

These questions all apply to the last month

The following statements describe the way in which asthma or shortness of breath or their treatment affect some people. Please tick the box that most closely applies to how you have felt over the last month

Selection of questions (13–32)	Not at all	Mildly	Moderately	Severely	Very severely
I have been troubled by episodes of shortness of breath	❑	❑	❑	❑	❑
I have been troubled by wheezing attacks	❑	❑	❑	❑	❑
I have been troubled by tightness in the chest	❑	❑	❑	❑	❑
I have been restricted in walking down the street on level ground or doing light housework because of asthma or shortness of breath	❑	❑	❑	❑	❑
I have been restricted in walking up hills or doing heavy housework because of asthma or shortness of breath	❑	❑	❑	❑	❑
I have felt tired or a general lack of energy	❑	❑	❑	❑	❑
I have been unable to sleep at night	❑	❑	❑	❑	❑
I have felt sad or depressed	❑	❑	❑	❑	❑
I have felt frustrated with myself	❑	❑	❑	❑	❑
I have felt anxious, under tension or stressed	❑	❑	❑	❑	❑
I have felt that asthma or shortness of breath is preventing me from achieving what I want from life					
Asthma or shortness of breath has interfered with my social life	❑	❑	❑	❑	❑
I have been limited in going to certain places because they are bad for my asthma	❑	❑	❑	❑	❑

continued

Selection of questions (13–32)	Not at all	Mildly	Moderately	Severely	Very severely
I have been limited in going to certain places because I have been afraid of getting an asthma attack and not being able to get help	❏	❏	❏	❏	❏
I have been restricted in the sports, hobbies or other recreations I can engage in because of my asthma or shortness of breath	❏	❏	❏	❏	❏
I have felt that asthma is controlling my life					
I have been worried about my present or future health because of asthma	❏	❏	❏	❏	❏
I have been worried about asthma shortening my life	❏	❏	❏	❏	❏
I have felt dependent on my asthma inhalers	❏	❏	❏	❏	❏

Who asks the questions

Survey is filled out by patients.

Time frame

Last month

Scoring system

Screening and treatment questions, mainly yes/no. Quality-of-life and severity questions: graded replies (eg not at all, mildly, moderately, severely, very severely). Each quality-of-life question is scored from 0 to 4, and the answers are then added together and scaled to give a quality-of-life score which lies between 0 (best; answers of 'none' to all questions) and 10 (worst; answers of 'very severely' to all questions). The square-root of this score has been shown to be approximately normally distributed.

Interpretation

Patients with more severe asthma had higher average AQLQ scores. No effect of the intervention on average AQLQ score (in patients in intervention practices compared with patients in control practices) was found.

SECTION FIVE
Bibliography

Ansted SJ, McDowell D, O'Driscoll BR (On behalf of START). The Salford Asthma Register — a mechanism for auditing a district asthma population and supporting GP asthma care (Abstract). *Thorax* 1998; **53**: A75

Ayriss MD, Bruins RH, Davidson M, Goel A, Kaleel MF. Improving asthma care through audit. *Eur Respir J* 1998; **12 (28)**: 282s

Barnes PJ. Inhaled glucocorticoids: new developments relevant to the updating of the asthma management guidelines. *Respir Med* 1996; **90**: 379–84

Barritt PW, Staples EB. Measuring success in asthma care: a repeat audit. *Brit J Gen Pract* 1991; **41**: 232–6

Beasley R, Cushley M, Holgate ST. A self management plan in the treatment of adult asthma. *Thorax* 1989; **44**: 200–4

Blackburn LA, Denn DJ, Oliver HF, Vickery PJM, Waldron J. One year's asthma admissions in Cornwall — still deficiencies in basic care. *Thorax* 1996; **51**: A62

Blaiss MS. Outcomes analysis in asthma. *J Am Med Assoc* 1997; **278(22)**: 1874–80

Bosley CM, Corden ZM, Cochrane GM. Psychosocial factors and asthma. *Respir Med* 1996; **90**: 453–7

British Thoracic Society and others. Guidelines on the management of asthma. *Thorax* 1993; **48**: S1–24

British Thoracic Association. Death from asthma in two regions of England. *Br Med J* 1982; **285**: 1251–5

Bryce FP, Neville RG, Crombie IK, Clark RA, McKenzie P. Controlled trial of an audit facilitator in diagnosis and treatment of childhood asthma in general practice. *Br Med J*. 1995; **310**: 838–42

Bucknall CE. Definitions of severity and outcome measures. *Respir Med* 1996; **90**: 447–52

Bucknall CE, Slack R, Godley C *et al*. Scottish Confidential Inquiry into Asthma Deaths 1994–96. *Eur Respir J* 1998; **12 (Suppl 28)**: 259s–60s.

Clough JB. Recommendations for peak flow monitoring in children. *Respir Med* 1996; **90**: 459–61

Connolly CK, Prescott RJ, Alcock SM, Gatnash AA. Actual over best function as an outcome measure in asthma. *Respir Med* 1994; **88**: 453–9

Cox BD, Huppert FA, Whichelow MJ eds. *The Health and Lifestyle Survey: seven years on*. Aldershot, 1993, Dartmouth: Dartmouth Publishing Company Ltd

Department of Health. *Asthma; an epidemiological overview*. London: HMSO, 1995

Department of Health. *Population Health Outcome Indicators for the NHS: a consultation document*. London: Department of Health, 1993

Dickinson J, Hutton S, Atkin A, Jones K. Reducing asthma morbidity in the community: the effect of a targeted nurse-run asthma clinic in an English general practice. *Respir Med* 1997; **91**: 634–40

Donabedian A. Evaluating the quality of medical care. *Millbank Memorial Fund Q* 1966; **44**: Suppl 166–206

Donnelly JE, Donnelly WJ, Thong YH. Parental perceptions and attitudes toward asthma and its treatment: a controlled study. *Soc Sci Med* 1987; **24**: 431–7

Douglas JWB, Ross JM. The effects of asthma on primary school performance. *Br J Educ Psychol* 1965; **35**: 28–40

Drummond N, Abdalla M, Beattie JAG, Buckingham JK, Lindsay T, Osman LM, Ross SJ, Russell I, Douglas JG, Legge JS, Friend JAR. Integrated care for asthma: a clinical social and economic evaluation. *Br Med J* 1994; **308**: 559–64

Duffy R, Neville RG, Hoskins G, Smith B, McCowan C. Who is admitted to hospital with asthma? *Asthma in General Practice* 1997; **5**: 5–7

Durham ST. Allergen avoidance measures. *Respir Med* 1996; **90**: 441–5

Fitzpatrick MF, Martin K, Fossey E *et al*. Snoring, asthma and sleep disturbance in Britain: a community-based survey. *Eur Respir J* 1993; **6**: 531–5

Gallup: *The Impact of Asthma Survey Results*, 1996. National Asthma Campaign. London: 1996

Grimshaw JM, Russell IT. Achieving health gain through clinical guidelines II: Ensuring guidelines change medical practice. *Qual Health Care* 1994; **3**: 45–52

Hall JM, Bennett M, Wagg A. The use of fluticasone propionate in the management of severe asthma in a general practice. *Thorax* 1995; **50**(Suppl 2): 6

Harrison BDW, Kelly, Y, Sodergren S, Willkes, Hyland M, Watkin SW. Attempts to assess asthma control in a hospital outpatient population. *Thorax* 1998; **53** (Suppl 4): A75

Hewer A. Outcome measures in stroke — a British view. *Stroke* Supplement II 1990; **21**(**9**): 52

Hill R, Williams J, Tattersfield A, Britton J. Change in the use of asthma as a diagnostic label for wheezing illness in schoolchildren. *Br Med J* 1989; **299**: 898

Holgate ST. Inhaled sodium cromoglycate. *Respir Med* 1996; **90**: 387–90

Holgate ST. The efficacy and therapeutic position of nedocromil sodium. *Respir Med* 1996; **90**: 391–4

Hopkins A. *Measuring the quality of medical care.* London: Royal College of Physicians, 1990

Hoskins G, Smith B, Neville RG, Clark RA. Does participation in distance learning and audit improve the care of patients with acute asthma attacks? *Health Bull* 1997; **55**: 150–5

Hoskins G, Smith B, Neville RG, Clark RA. The Tayside Asthma Management Initiative. *Health Bull* 1998; **56**: 586–91

Hyland ME, Crocker GR. Validation of an asthma quality of life diary in a clinical trial. *Thorax* 1995; **50**: 724–30

Jeffrey M, Meadows K, Greene T and Jeffrey AA. Results of a postal questionnaire. *Thorax* 1996; **51**: 62

Jones K. Asthma — still a challenge for general practice. *J Roy Coll Gen Pract* 1989; **39**: 254–6

Jones K, Cleary R, Hyland M. Predictive value of a simple asthma morbidity index in a general practice population. *Br J Gen Pract* 1999; **49**: 23–6

Jones KP, Bain DJG, Middleton M, Mullee MA. Correlates of asthma morbidity in primary care. *Br Med J* 1992; **304**: 361–4

Jones KP, Charleton IH, Middleton M, Preece WJ, Hill AP. Targeting asthma care in general practice using a morbidity index. *Br Med J* 1992; **304**: 1353–6

Jones KP, Mullee MA. Proactive, nurse-run asthma care in general practice reduces asthma morbidity: scientific fact or medical assumption? *Br J Gen Pract* 1995; **45**: 497–9

Jones PW. Quality of Life measurement in asthma. *Eur Respir J* 1995; **8**: 885–7

Jones KP, Mullee MA, Middleton M, Chapman E, Holgate ST. Peak flow based asthma self-management: A randomised controlled study in general practice. *Thorax* 1995; **50**: 851–7

Juniper EF, Guyatt GH, Epstein RS, Ferrie PJ, Jaeschke R, Hiller TK. Evaluation of impairment of health related quality of life in asthma: development of a questionnaire for use in clinical trials. *Thorax* 1992; **47**: 76–83

Katz PP, Yelin EH, Smith S, Blanc PD. Perceived control of asthma: development and validation of a questionnaire. *Am J Respir Crit Care Med* 1997; **155**: 577–82

Keeley D. How to achieve better outcome in treatment of asthma in general practice. *Br Med J* 1993; **307**: 1261–3

Lahdensuo A, Haahtela T, Herrala J, Kava T *et al.* Randomised comparison of guided self management and traditional treatment of asthma over one year. *Br Med J* 1996; **312**: 748–52

Lahdensuo A, Haahtela T, Herrala J, Kava T *et al.* Randomised comparison of cost effectiveness of guided self management and traditional treatment of asthma in Finland. *Br Med J* 1998; **316**: 1138–9

Lenney W, Wells NEJ, O'Neill BA. The burden of paediatric asthma. *Eur Respir Rev* 1994; **4**: 49–62

Madge P, McColl J, Paton J. Impact of a nurse-led home management training programme in children admitted to hospital with acute asthma: a randomised controlled trial. *Thorax* 1997; **52**: 223–8

Marks GB, Burney PG, Premaratne UN, Simpson J, Webb J. Asthma in Greenwich, UK: impact of the disease and current management practices. *Eur Respir J* 1997; **10**: 1224–9

Martin AJ, Landau LI, Phelan PD. Asthma from childhood at age 21: the patient and his disease. *Br Med J* 1982; **284**: 380–2

Mathur R, Clark RA, Dhillon DP, Winter JH, Lipworth BJ. Re-audit of acute asthma admissions using a severity marker stamp and determinants of an outcome measure. *Scott Med J* 1997; **42**: 49–52

McColl AJ, Gulliford MC. *Population Health Outcome Indicators of the NHS: a feasibility study for the Department of Health.* London: Faculty of Public Health Medicine of the Royal College of Physicians, 1993

McColl E, Steen IN, Meadows KA, Hutchinson A, Eccles MP, Hewison J, Fowler P, Blades SM. Developing outcome measures for ambulatory care — an application to asthma and diabetes. *Soc Sci Med* 1995; **41**: 1339–48

McCowan C, Neville RG, Crombie IK, Clark RA, Warner FC. The facilitator effect: results from a four-year follow-up of children with asthma. *Br J Gen Pract* 1997; **47**: 156–60

National Centre for Health Outcomes Development. *Asthma.* Report of a working group to the Department of Health. London: NCHOD, 1999

Neville R. Two approaches to effective asthma audit. *Practitioner* 1995; **239**: 203–5

Neville R. Patient education and guided self management plans. *Respir Med* 1996; **90**: 385–6

Neville RG, Hoskins G, Smith B, Clark RA. Observations on the structure, process and clinical outcomes of asthma care in general practice. *Br J Gen Pract* 1996; **46**: 583–7

Nocon A, Booth T. The social impact of asthma. *Family Practice* 1991; **8**: 37–41

Office of Health Economics. *Compendium of Health Statistics,* 10th Edition. London: OHE, 1997

Office for National Statistics. *New Earnings Survey Labour Market Trends.* London: ONS, November 1997

Osman LM, Abdalla MI, Beattie JAG *et al* (GRASSIC) Reducing hospital admission through computer supported education for asthma patients. *Br Med J* 1994; **308**: 568–71

Osman LM, Russell IT, Fiddes J, Friend JAR, Legge JS, Douglas JG. Integrated care for asthma : matching care to the patient. *Eur Respir J* 1996; **9**: 444–8

Peckham C, Butler N. A national study of asthma in childhood. *J Epidemiol Commun Health* 1978; **32**: 79–85

Premaratne UN, Sterne JAC, Marks GB, Webb JR, Azima H, Burney PGJ. Clustered randomised trial of an intervention to improve the management of asthma: Greenwhich Asthma Study. *Br Med J* 1999; **318**: 1251–5

Price DB. Patterns of prescribing of inhaled steroids over a seven year period in a general practice and its implications. *Thorax* 1995; **50**: 443P

Price DB, Appleby JL. Fluticasone propionate: an audit of outcomes and cost effectiveness in primary care. *Respir Med* 1998; **92**: 351–3

Price DB, Cargill K, Wolfe S, Darby H. Salmetorol xinafoate: an analysis of outcomes and cost effectiveness using a primary care database. *Respir Med* 1998; **92**: 1302–4

Price D, Ryan D. *Asthma: The Key Facts,* Middlesex: Allen & Hanburys, 1998

Rimington LD, Aaronovsky L, Mowatt A, Wharburton E, Ryland I, Pearson MG. Use of a simple patient focused asthma morbidity score. *Eur Respir J* 1997; **10**: 194s

Robertson R, Osman LM, Douglas JG. Adult asthma review in general practice : nurses' perception of their role. *Family Practice* 1997; **14**: 227–32

Royal College of General Practitioners, Office of Population Censuses and Surveys, and Department of Health. *Morbidity Statistics from General Practice, Fourth National Study 1991–92.* London: HMSO 1995

Santanello NC, Barber BL, Reiss TF, Friedman BS, Juniper EF, Zhang J. Measurement characteristics of two asthma symptom diary scales for use in clinical trials. *Eur Respir J* 1997; **10**: 646–51

Secretary of State for Health. *The New NHS* London: Stationary Office, 1997.

Slack R, Bucknall CE. Re-admission rates are associated with differences in the process of care in acute asthma. *Qual Health Care* 1997; **6**: 194–8

Smith DH, Malone DC, Lawson KA *et al.* A national estimate of the economic costs of asthma. *Am J Respir Crit Care Med* 1997; **156**: 787–93

Steen N, Hutchinson A, McColl E, Eccles MP *et al.* Development of a symptom-based outcome measure for asthma. *Br Med J* 1994; **309**: 1065–8

Waldron J, Denn DJ, Oliver HF, Vickery PJM, Waldron MJ, Blackburn LA. *A questionnaire to assess the link between asthma patients, their knowledge about management and their feelings about their illness.* Cornwall Heathcare Trust, Asthma Information Centre

Worrall G, Chaulk P, Freake D. The effects of clinical practice guidelines on patient outcomes in primary care: a systematic review. *Can Med Assoc J.* 1997; **157**: 642